Becoming a Mother

BECOMING A MOTHER

. . .

From Birth to Six Months

Gro Nylander
M.D., Ph.D.
*Senior consultant in Obstetrics and Gynecology,
the National Hospital, University of Oslo, Norway*

Photography by Herdis Maria Siegert

Celestial Arts
Berkeley / Toronto

To my elder son, Olav,
who taught me the most about being a mom.

A Kirsty Melville Book

Celestial Arts
P.O. Box 7123
Berkeley, California 94707
www.tenspeed.com

Distributed in Australia by Simon and Schuster Australia, in Canada by Ten Speed Press
Canada, in New Zealand by Southern Publishers Group, in South Africa by Real Books,
in Southeast Asia by Berkeley Books, and in the United Kingdom and Europe
by Airlift Book Company.

Cover Design by Betsy Stromberg
Interior Design by Tasha Hall

Library of Congress Cataloging-in-Publication Data
Nylander, Gro.
Becoming a mother / Gro Nylander.
p. ; cm.
"A Kirsty Melville book."
Originally published: [Oslo] : Gyldendal Norsk, c2000.
Includes bibliographical references and index.
ISBN 1-58761-131-7
1. Pregnancy—Psychological aspects. 2. Childbirth—Psychological aspects.
3. Infants—Care. 4. Mother and child. 5. Motherhood. 6. Mothers.
[DNLM: 1. Infant Care—Popular Works. 2. Breast Feeding—Popular Works.
3. Postnatal Care—Popular Works. WS 113 B398 2002]   I. Title.
RG556 .N95 2002
618.2'0019—dc21
                                                    2002007454

First printing, 2002

Printed in the United States of America

1 2 3 4 5 6 7 8 9 10 — 05 04 03 02

Contents

Thank you!

Many young parents have read all or part of this manuscript and have given useful responses along the way: Mona and Jan Peter, Nina and George, Mette and Paul Espen, Sally and Per, Elisabeth and Lars, Eli, Ragnhild, and Kjersti and Haavard.

All the parents we asked willingly said yes to being photographed with their babies by photographer Herdis Maria Siegert, who did outstanding work.

Midwives Anne Kaasen and Nina Nylander, pediatrician Ingrid Helland, and healthcare nurse and international board-certified lactation consultant Elisabeth Tufte read the first draft of the book and made valuable, professional contributions.

Professors Per Brandtzaeg, Lorentz Irgens, Asbjørn Langslet, Trond Markestad, and Torleiv Rognum; veterinary surgeon Bergljot Børresen; and Nina Øyen, M.D., have quality-assured individual parts with their extensive expertise.

Editor Jorunn Borthen Gundersen has led me through the labyrinth of writing this book.

My own family has, as always, been a great joy and inspiration. My daughter and medical student, Astrid, has read the whole manuscript and given useful advice.

I hope that because of the support of all these contributors, *Becoming a Mother* will be so interesting that you will use this book even if you don't like reading parenting books, so rich in content that you will learn something even if you are experienced, and so technically correct that you will find it useful even if you are a healthcare professional.

Gro Nylander
Høvik, 2002

Introduction

DEAR NEW MOM

One important reason for writing about the time after birth is that the people of the Western world currently lack support from the traditional neighbors of bygone days. Our foremothers had familiar, experienced women around them to help during labor. Afterward, these women cared for the new mother and baby, helping them to get started at breastfeeding. If there were problems, they had the experience of generations to draw on. In the postpartum period, they did the women's work, cared for older children, kept house, and even fed—and milked—the farm animals. Others came bringing food and delicacies to keep the new mother well nourished.

A FELLOWSHIP OF WOMEN

This sisterhood is still seen in other cultures, where a new baby is a sensation and cause for rejoicing by all, where grandmothers, aunts, and sisters can't do enough for the new mother the first days and weeks after birth. They listen to the story of the birth and tell about their own birth experiences, feed the new mother nourishing meals, massage her belly, and give her and the baby plenty of tender loving care. This sisterhood still exists in our society, too, in some areas. But far too often, new mothers are newcomers to where they live and have no family or close friends nearby—or those they do have are too busy. A new mother often ends up at home alone with her baby. No wonder she feels insecure, tired, and at times a bit abandoned. It is hardly an advantage for a new mother to be on her own with her baby most of the time.

DAD IS IMPORTANT, TOO

Do you think I've forgotten the father? Not at all! A baby is not the only one who is born, as the saying goes; a mother is born, too—and a father as well, if you ask me. Today, fathers are most often present at the birth and are actively involved with the baby in a completely different way than were fathers of past generations. This is terrific, and this book is also meant for fathers. But the new father is also inexperienced and new to his role. And no matter how good a father he is, he will still return to work after a short paternity leave and may be gone for large parts of the day.

GRANDPARENTS

Today's grandmothers are often part of the paid workforce. They also belong to a generation that breastfed very little. This was not because they didn't want to breastfeed—nearly all of them tried—but rigid hospital routines got in the way. Breastfeeding often turned out to be a fiasco, because mothers were taught to offer the breast far too seldom and for too short a time. In the 1960s, only about 20 percent of babies continued to receive breast milk at the age of three months. Today that figure is around 90 percent. Grandma would love to help, but she doesn't always have good experience to pass on. And besides, she has her job. On the other hand, grandfathers often volunteer as baby-sitters these days, something that was uncommon in the past.

MY OWN EXPERIENCE AS A MOTHER

I have given birth to three children; my firstborn was disabled. We struggled through a difficult and short period of breastfeeding. I saw with amazement that my engorged breasts from the hospital disappeared, and I was advised to skip every other meal at the breast to save up enough milk for the next meal. At six weeks, my son weighed the same as he had weighed at birth. I gave up and brooded and searched for more knowledge. Breastfeeding improved with each succeeding child. With increased knowledge, security, and networking, I became a breastfeeding peer counselor and eventually a physician. I have worked with mothers and babies for several decades.

My Work as an Obstetrician

I have been an obstetric specialist for more than twenty-five years and am still deeply moved by each and every birth. But I also see what a test of strength lies in birth and during the time just after, physically and emotionally. Sometimes a new mother is dismayed when she is not overwhelmed by happiness and love for her baby right away. We live in a time when childbirth is romanticized so that the birth itself is supposed to be the great happening in the young couple's life. Mother- and father-to-be prepare and plan carefully. They forget that the body most often gets through labor by itself. They can't do much about it one way or the other, despite courses and books. They are often unprepared for the time just after birth, however, and this period is what psychologists describe as a life crisis.

The Start of the Mother-Child Relationship

This important phase can start a positive cycle that will influence both mother and child for the rest of their lives. We all know that it is easy to like someone who shows they like us. Every time I do the rounds in the postnatal ward, I learn something about this bond. I personally know all the mothers, babies, and fathers whose stories are in this book. Most are presented under their own names. Some have been given aliases because I haven't asked their permission or because their stories are sensitive.

Working for Breastfeeding

Over many years, I have been concerned about breastfeeding and parental interaction with the newborn child. The fervor from the pioneer days of Ammehjelpen, the Norwegian breastfeeding mothers' association, has followed me throughout my professional life. First on my own, and later with capable colleagues in the Baby-Friendly Hospital Initiative, I traveled to many parts of the world to update health workers so they would improve their skills in helping mothers with their breastfeeding. Because this activity has led to a fair amount of media exposure, I get many questions from new parents. I never have enough time to answer all of them. That is one reason I finally agreed to write a book about the period after birth, five years after the suggestion was first made.

Early Discharge from the Hospital

Another reason to put my experience, knowledge, and feelings down on paper is that insurance companies and hospitals have discovered a new way to save money: by discharging mothers and new babies early from the hospital.

Several decades ago, much was done wrong with the best of intentions—but at least the postpartum stay then was a kind of vacation for a week or two. The new mother was pampered and cared for like a queen, even though her heart often ached at being kept apart from her baby.

Now the mother has got her baby back, and never have so many women in Norway breastfed for so long, at least in this century. Ironically, however, while the new mother is with her baby and generally enjoys this, current trends and cuts in services mean that she is nearly exhausted because she must manage on her own.

Remember, the single thing that only a mother can do is breastfeed. Even so, it is expected in many wards that a new mother change diapers, care for herself, fetch her meals, carry her dirty dishes, make her bed, and water the flowers she's been given. She needs to make it to exercise sessions, debrief with her midwife, attend a breastfeeding class and the pediatrician's examinations, and learn infant care—all in the course of just a few days. Many women are placed directly in a "patient hotel" two hours after birth. There, even fewer staff are available to care for them.

The trend of seeing birth as a natural event and the new mother as a healthy woman, in itself a positive trend, has led to shorter hospital stays. The new mother is usually sent home a few days after birth whether she wants to leave or not. This is fine for women whose pregnancies and births have been straightforward, whose babies are calm, and whose milk flows freely. It is fine when mother and baby come home to a pleasant situation and good care, or when health services follow up with home-based care.

Going home early is worse for the mother when things aren't so good. When she doesn't have anyone to ask for advice—when her stitches are aching, when she is still bleeding, when her breasts feel as hard as rocks, with nipples like open sores, when the baby just cries, when perspiration and baby blues tears are equally voluminous—the responsibility seems unbearable, and the new mother has only a vague memory of sleeping at night.

This is a book about joy and wonder and the cleverness of nature. But it is also a book to help women during a time that for many is the toughest in their lives—as brand new mothers.

Despite the equality of the sexes, we must not forget that it is the woman who gets pregnant, carries and nourishes the fetus, gives birth to the baby with joy and pain, and feeds the baby at her breast. This is biology. No one can take these things away from you as a childbearing woman or do them for you. Therefore, this book is addressed most of all to you, Dear New Mom, to help you help yourself.

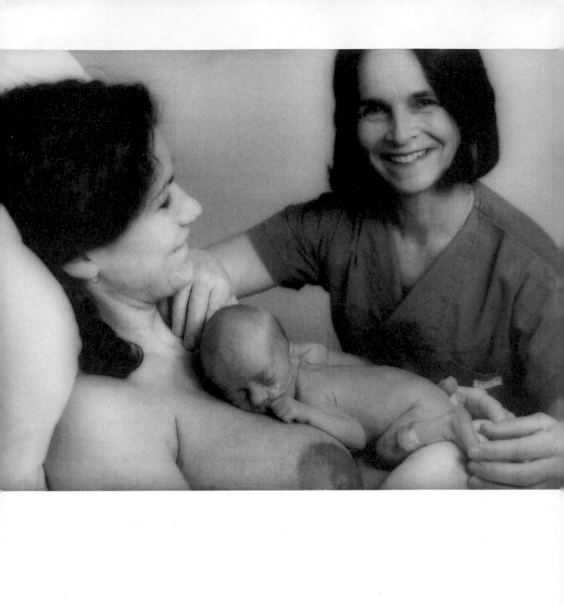

Chapter 1

From Womb to Breast: Newborn and Determined

Little Frances has just been born in delivery room 3. Would you like to come in and join me very quietly in a corner to admire what happens right afterward?

Frances has everything in her favor for a good start at life outside the womb. She is a much-longed-for baby, and her mother, Ann, has had a good labor and birth. It took fourteen hours, and it hurt, but it progressed well and was bearable. The neck of Ann's womb opened steadily, and there were good intervals between contractions. Ann rested so well during the pauses that she managed with no pain relief. She spent some time in a warm bath when things were at their most intense, right before the womb was fully open. In the breaks between her pushing contractions, she even slept. Those contractions weren't painful. "They were like rafting," she said later. They were violent natural forces that took hold of her. She just had to hang on and help with all her might. She was massaged around the opening of her birth canal with warm oil, and the tissue had time to stretch gradually.

Frances slid out slowly, slippery as a fish, without giving her mom so much as a tear.

Now she lies there, between Ann's legs: small, damp, strange, and a bit bloody. Warm, gloved hands hold her, wipe her nose and mouth carefully, dry her hair. Her cord pulsates powerfully, because the placenta is still providing nutrition and oxygen from Ann to her baby. Frances lies lower than Ann for a few minutes. This is fine, because now Frances gets her last blood transfusion from her mother before she continues on perhaps the most important journey of her life: the journey from womb to breast.

Frances is bluish and greasy with vernix. She squeaks at first, then finally cries. The helpers smile. Joe, the father—for that is what he suddenly has become—sits down with a bump and a relieved groan. Tired and satisfied, Ann senses that now it is all over. All the long months of waiting, the contractions, the thrill of the final phase when she pushed, the burning sensation of her pelvic floor—finally over.

First Encounter

The midwife hands the infant to Ann. She is now a mother for the first time. Mom. She senses this, and she senses her baby.

Someone has unbuttoned Ann's shirt. Frances lies naked on Ann's chest and belly, and a nurse gives Ann a warm towel so she can dry off her baby herself. Rubbing gently, Ann gets her baby dry and warm and stimulates her breathing, encourages her to keep on living. Her actions resemble the thorough licking and nudging that other mammals give their newborn offspring. A bit clumsily, Ann handles Frances, who gradually turns pink as she lies on her mom's belly. The big, warm belly has suddenly collapsed, with lots of room for the baby on top. Joe cuts the cord where the midwife points. A bit shaky and with a lump in his throat, he separates daughter from mother. Frances has become *his* daughter as well.

Frances cries a little, tenses her body restlessly, and doesn't seem at all happy to be out of the cozy cave of the womb, where she lived for nine months. Under the heating lamp above the bed, she can lie naked, move freely, touch, and be touched. Ann begins hesitantly to handle her baby, with light, cautious fingertips. She becomes more sure of herself, feels the infant's hands and feet, pats the small limbs, strokes the back with her hand, holds tenderly, rocks her baby a bit.

It is right that Ann's hands should be the first to touch Frances without gloves. Frances has been virtually free of bacteria in the womb. Now her entire skin will be covered with bacteria. Most of them are benign, but some are unfriendly. That is why it is important that the first ones come from Ann; she will produce antibodies in her milk against these bacteria and thereby protect Frances. The next person to touch the baby might well be her dad, Joe. A couple living together have many bacterial strains in common, so a mother's milk protects most often even against bacteria from the father—and from the rest of the family.

"I See You"

Frances settles down and lies still. She opens her dark eyes to squint. She has enormous pupils that seem to be looking into infinity. Ann moves Frances a bit to see her well, bends her head toward Frances, looks into her eyes: "She sees me!" Some researchers have found that early eye contact is important to strengthening the bond with a new baby. One thing is certain—the newborn will normally gaze and gaze and will prefer to stare at a face with shining eyes over anything else.

Frances fusses a little again, stretches her legs, flexes them well, kicks off, and slides slightly upward. Then she rests.

"Listen to Me"

Frances starts to appeal to her mom with small, sharp sounds: "Eh! Eh!" Ann answers, without consciously thinking about doing so. With a soft, high-pitched voice, she says, "My little girl. You're here at last. How wonderful! Little Treasure, we've been waiting for you. Hi, Sweetheart!" It is baby talk in a silken voice. Ann's precious maternal instincts cause her to raise the pitch of her voice this way without further reflection. Most women do this when they speak to an infant. It's a smart occurrence: research has shown that babies show interest in just this pitch of voice, whereas a deep voice, no matter how loving, seldom captivates them the same way. Research also shows that babies prefer the voice of their own mother over that of anyone else, surely because the baby is used to that voice from the womb. A father who has spoken a lot or sung songs close to the belly comes a close second.

Ann and the newborn Frances continue to chat undisturbed. Joe sits with them; with his arm around Ann's shoulders, he embraces them both. Ann holds the baby; Joe holds the woman who has become the mother of their child. It is his family, the family unit, but his time for direct contact with Frances is not just yet.

Frances bends her arm, brings her hand to her face, flings out her hand, stretches, flexes her fingers. Something stimulates the grasp reflex in her palm: a convenient nipple, her father's finger. She grips strongly . . . holds . . . loses her grasp . . . calls again: "Eh! Eh!" Calm settles over the room. The helpers quietly watch and wait, tidying up in the background.

The afterbirth comes, fills the birth canal, and requires only a little push before it is delivered. It is big, soft, and glossy with the translucent sac in which Frances has lain. Once key to Frances's survival, it has now lost its importance.

"Mmm—Smells Good"

Ann sniffs, greedily seeking the scent of the baby's head. She does not know that this is how nearly all women smell babies. After a few days, many mothers in one study managed to find their own babies while blindfolded, by scent alone. In fact, even sensually blunted modern humans are more aware of scents than most people realize. Smell is important for animals other than humans as well. A ewe that has just given birth will not allow a lamb to approach her udder until she has first sniffed the lamb. Animals that live in groups sniff the newborn carefully as soon as the mother permits it.

Frances uses her tiny nose, too. The dark area around Ann's nipple, the areola, is covered with glands that produce oils to protect against moisture and injury but that also smell attractive to the baby and lead it in the right direction. In one study, researchers washed one breast of each participating new mother well with soap just after birth but made sure that both breasts were warm and dry when the baby was placed on the mother's belly. When the babies were given time to search on their own, most of them found their way to the unwashed breast and started to suckle there. Clearly, Mom does not need to bathe immediately after birth; she is meant to have a scent.

Ann takes in the smell, the sound, and the sight of her baby. She nuzzles and cuddles and nearly tastes Frances, her lips against the damp, downy hair. Ann does not realize that this process of bonding with the baby resembles the process that all other mammals go through as well. Scents are dispersed and enhanced. Perhaps Ann's moist kissing parallels the licking of other mammal mothers?

Searching

Suddenly Frances catches sight of the dark nipple and areola. Her eyes open wide in fascination. Is it recorded somewhere in her mind that she must pursue this pleasant formation?

Just afterward, Frances's mouth starts to move. Her lips open and shut and stretch to the side in a grimace, a searching half smile. Her tongue emerges and touches her lips, licks a little; she drools. But nothing comes inside her longing mouth—yet. She has to keep working. She snorts a little fluid out her nose, grunts, and struggles. She feels a nipple tickling her on one cheek. Her rooting reflex is aroused; she tries to turn toward that breast more and more. This same thing may be observed in any healthy newborn. Babies in cribs away from their mothers twist desperately toward anything that touches their cheeks: a blanket, a friendly hand, the chest of a blushing father who tries to stand in for mother while they wait for her together.

At last Frances lifts her head straight up from where she lies on Ann's belly to search with her mouth. She wavers. Her head is too heavy; she falls down on her other cheek. She rests again, cries, lifts once more, sways, and misses. Perhaps it would be easier for Frances if Ann were more upright and held her? Then Frances would need only to search from side to side and would not have to hold her heavy head on her thin neck.

Research shows that apes must learn to breastfeed. The birth usually goes well. The chimp mother manages on her own and actually assists the baby out with her hands. She lifts up the baby and licks the young chimp's face—and behind—clean. But after that, she apparently has no real notion of what to do. That is where the baby comes in. As with humans, the newborn chimp's voice gives the mother an irresistible order to do something. Each time the baby squeaks, the mother chimp moves the young one around on her body, seemingly without purpose. One series of photos shows a new chimp mother in exasperation, even placing the baby on top of her own head. At last she finds a place where the baby settles, namely, the place where the young chimp finds something to suckle. Next time, they find this place a little more quickly. The baby gives the signals, roots, and works at it, and the mother helps out.

Despite the large brains of humans and everything those brains allow us—abstract thought, formal schooling, complex societies, space travel—we are closely related to the large primates biologically. Humans have more genetic material in common with chimpanzees, in fact, than Indian elephants have with African elephants. Like other primates, human females are driven to a large degree during birth and the time immediately following by instincts and hormones. As long as the hormones are given the opportunity to work, they help mother and baby during and just after birth.

Decades ago, doctors as well as parents commonly believed newborn babies to be completely helpless. We did not believe that they could see well, control their gaze, feel pain, lift their head, or turn. Today we know that they are capable of all these things from birth and have an impressive amount of inborn knowledge. Their first and most important goal is to reach the mother's breast. Their instincts tell them that suckling at the breast will ensure their survival.

Encouraged by her mother's soft, high-pitched voice as it soothes and inspires her, and by warm hands that hold her, Frances begins again. Now, perhaps? There. She lands with the nipple nearly in her mouth. She flares her mouth toward it, turns her head a bit more, opens wide as a baby bird—no, as a searching baby human. She licks and sucks at her mother's skin, smacks her tongue. She extends her tongue as far as she can, forms it into a U–shape. Her mouth opens wider and wider, nearly desperate. There! She reaches her goal! Hungrily, her lips close around a large mouthful of breast. Nearly all the pigmented skin of the areola has vanished. Frances suckles as though her life depended on it—and indeed it does.

Helpers are nearby; they adjust Frances's position to bring her nearer to her mother. At last, Ann and Frances are lying close, directly facing each other with their whole bodies. Frances's chin is pressed against her mother's breast. Her lips are flanged outward, and the suckling action can be seen right back to her ears. Frances's wide-open mouth ensures that the breast reaches all the way to her soft palate and triggers the powerful suckling reflex. Healthy babies given time to complete this searching process after birth—uninterrupted by weighing, bathing, or being dressed—rarely have problems taking the breast correctly.

Surging Hormones

When Frances nurses, sensory impulses travel from Ann's breasts to her spinal cord and from there to her brain and her pituitary gland. This tiny hormone factory immediately starts to release breastfeeding hormones into Ann's circulation. The hormones are pumped through all her arteries and received by every cell in her body. Now, just after birth, oxytocin is the most important hormone. It must reach the organs where the receptor systems have been alerted by the birth. Birth attendants can give a synthetic version of this hormone if needed, during and after birth, but what a convenience it is when the home-made variety does its job!

The womb is one of the organs alerted by birth. It contracts strongly when oxytocin flows in response to the baby's suckling. The muscular uterine walls expel the afterbirth and stop the flow of blood, preventing abnormal bleeding. The breast is another target organ for oxytocin—perhaps the most important. Even the smallest mammary gland is surrounded by a network of smooth muscle cells. When oxytocin reaches these cells, they contract rapidly and squeeze the milk in the glands outward to the nipple.

Frances gets only a few drops for all her energetic suckling just after birth. The amount is scarcely measurable, but it calms her and initiates the almost magical effect of breast milk. Oxytocin controls the important milk-ejection reflex, which in time will make milk drip and even stream out if Ann so much as thinks about Frances.

In addition, oxytocin works on Ann's brain. In laboratory animals, oxytocin has been shown to lead to increased interest in and care for newborn offspring. If given oxytocin, a rat with no young—even a male rat—starts to build a nest and may even kidnap the young of other rats and cuddle them. Humans are driven by many things besides hormones, but perhaps oxytocin helps Ann to get started at being a mother. After all, hormones strongly influence humans in other phases of life, as in the premenstrual cycle of some women.

Now, after Frances has sucked for a while, Ann feels a comfortable drowsiness and increased well-being. The whole family relaxes together after an intense effort. Left to themselves, Ann, Joe, and Frances enjoy this quiet time alone together.

DAD STANDS GUARD

Joe has yet to hold his baby daughter; so far, he has only patted her tentatively. He is, however, intensely preoccupied with mother and child. He sits with them, embraces them, comments on their activities, stands guard. The door opens; the shift has changed and a new nurse appears. Joe stares, irritated, almost aggressive, and leans over his family. Has the birth stimulated some protective instincts in him? It

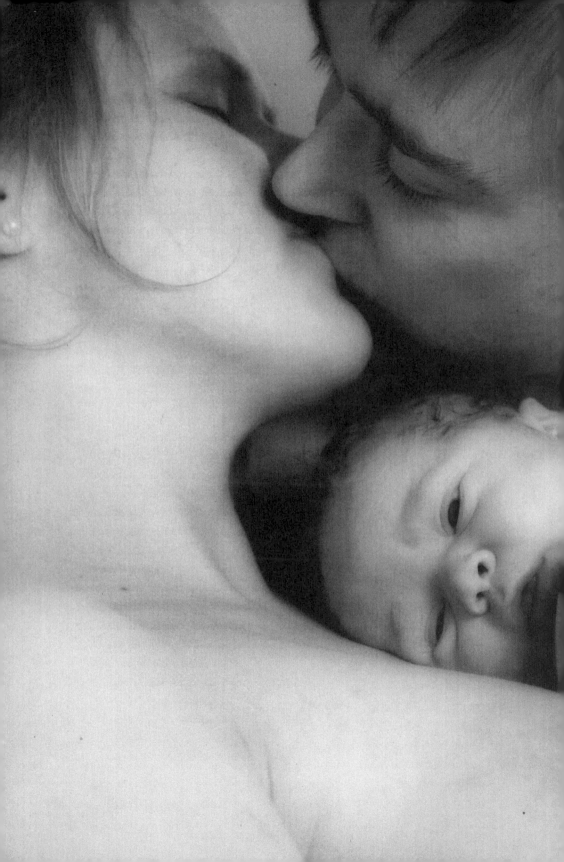

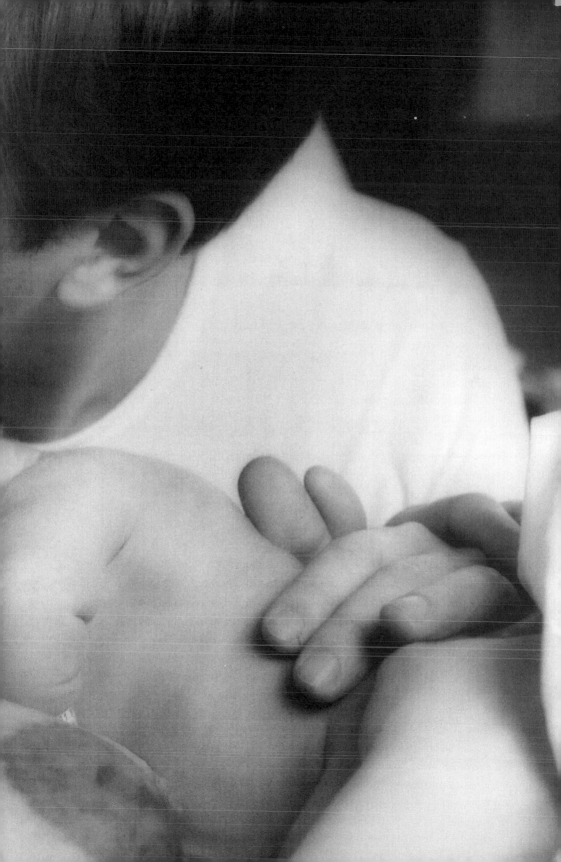

can often appear so in new fathers. Joe has become what I call a "daddy lion."

We tiptoe out of our observation post in the corner of the room. We now know that all of this is typical after birth: this path from womb to breast. It is a process that usually takes from thirty to sixty minutes—but it could take significantly less or more time. Some babies cry a lot or have to rest frequently during this time. Others need help finding the breast, particularly if the mother has received pain-relief medication such as pethidine (Demerol), which can temporarily dull the baby's feeding reflexes. However long it takes, though, the process is repeated, in about the same order, by most healthy, full-term babies—when conditions allow. This activity—this business of starting breastfeeding—is a small, consummate, everyday miracle.

On the path from womb to breast, the baby:

- Most often shows crawling movements by bending and stretching the hips and knees.

- Stretches and bends the arms.

- Brings one hand to the face, and gradually to the mouth.

- Grasps at anything that touches the palms.

- Calls out to the mother with small, high-pitched, sharp "Eh! Eh!" cries.

- Listens attentively to the mother, who talks in a "baby" voice.

- Regards the mother's face, especially her eyes.

- Sniffs and breathes loudly at the mother's breast.

- Begins to move the lips, showing rooting movements.

- Sticks the tongue out and drools.

- Attempts to turn the head toward anything that touches the cheek.

- Turns the head quickly from side to side "in a rooting movement."

- Opens the mouth wide when the nipple or anything else touches the lips.

- Forms the tongue into a U–shaped cup before taking the breast into the mouth.

· · ·

CHAPTER 2

Putting Yourself in Your Baby's Place

At times I wonder if the desperate cry of a newborn baby conveys approximately this message: "Help! I am terrified and freezing cold. The light is hurting my eyes, and all the noises frighten me. I feel exhausted and half suffocated after that journey. I am straining to get enough oxygen, in a completely new way. You must be forgetting that I am used to lying in muted, red darkness and only hearing distant sounds as I am surrounded by soft walls and my lovely, warm waters."

Being born is an intense experience. We don't remember how it feels, but it is possible to fantasize about it. Toward the end of pregnancy, less and less space is available inside the womb. The dancing about, from the time when there was proper elbow room, is over. There is hardly room for a real kick. The experience is more like moving inside a narrow sleeping bag. During the contractions of labor itself, the uterus squeezes firmly around the baby. The baby is driven and pressed forth. Then the infant emerges in a boundless world, arms and legs flailing far out from the body.

French obstetrician Frederic Leboyer attracted attention with his book *Birth without Violence,* published in the 1970s. He calls the newborn's facial expression "the mask of terror." We often laugh in relief in the delivery room when the baby screams. Leboyer compared this screaming to the expressions of victims of torture. Although the analogy may be a bit strong, if you study the photograph of a wailing newborn and accept Leboyer's comparison, your smile may grow shaky.

Leboyer claims that birth is an enormous trauma for the baby, psychologically as well as physically. Psychotherapist Stanislav Grof agrees and claims to be able to take adults back to fetal life and their own births. He describes the happy existence of the fetus in contrast to the "no-way-out hell" of the first stage of labor. When finally born, the baby experiences "a deep perception of spiritual liberation, deliverance, and salvation." Grof believes that this tremendous trial, followed by the victory of emerging into the light, is positive for the individual's subsequent spiritual development.

Most of us probably find it difficult to have any definite opinions on this sort of thing. The one thing that is certain is that the newborn baby does calm down when comforted. But how can we best ease the transition?

"Don't Frighten Me with Noise"

In the womb, the baby has listened to sounds for many months, but those sounds have been muted by the waters, the walls of the uterus, and the mother's body. During labor, the baby may hear new sounds from the mother. After birth, there are loud voices, the jangling of metallic instruments, shouts, and laughter. Perhaps this is all quite terrifying. In any case, it is striking how many newborns calm down when they have arrived on their mother's belly and chest. Suddenly they hear something familiar again: the soft, rhythmic beat of the mother's heart in a well-known tempo; the sound of the mother's lungs filling and emptying as the baby is rocked in movements reminiscent of the rocking inside the womb.

Many years ago, I heard a researcher explain that he had investigated the effects of different types of music on the fetal heartbeat. It turned out that the heart beat faster when traditional folk fiddle music was played near the uterus than when slow, classical music was played. This was no big surprise, perhaps. Newer studies have shown that the baby recognizes not only the mother's voice, but also familiar songs heard often from within the womb before birth. The mother's voice sounds different when the sound is transmitted through air, but it is still hers.

Often the mother first begins to talk to her baby when the baby asks for her. Perhaps the little "Eh? Eh?" of the baby is really to say, "Hi, Mom! Talk to me, because I am scared and confused. What is it really like out here? Hold me tight. Carefully, because being touched is new to me. And stroke me softly. First on my arms and legs, because they

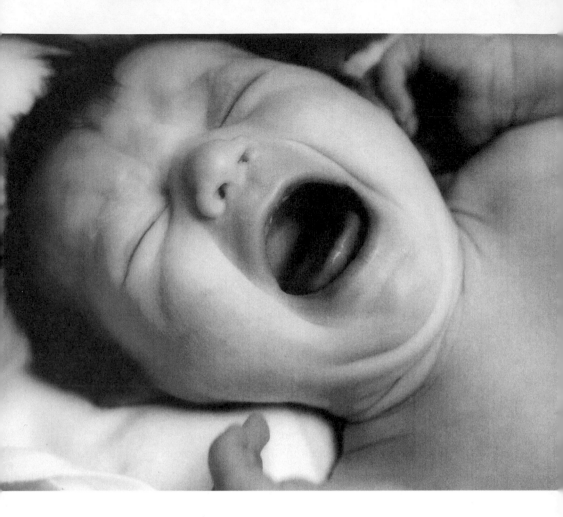

know you well. Then my back, because that is what I am used to rubbing against the womb. But my soft belly has been protected in the fetal position. Wait a bit before you touch me there."

You can almost imagine that the mother senses this message. Most new mothers seem to instinctively follow approximately these "guidelines" when handed their baby for the first time.

"LET ME SMELL YOU"

The baby has still more to say. "Mmmm . . . What smells so delightful—familiar, and at the same time so new and attractive? I simply must get it into my mouth. Don't run off to the shower now, Mom, before

I have reached my goal in peace and quiet. And sniff me, too! Right now, before anyone has washed me with soap."

The baby recognizes the scent of the mother's skin, even though most smelling up until now has been of amniotic fluid. The most irresistible scent, though, is that of breast milk. A baby given the choice between the scent of his or her mother's skin without milk and the scent of another woman's milk will opt for the milk.

In most mammals, scent is an essential determinant of bonding between mother and child. This has been especially well investigated in sheep. If a ewe doesn't get to sniff her lamb within an hour of birth, she won't have anything to do with the lamb later. This bonding through scent appears to be influenced by the hormone oxytocin, which is present in very high concentrations during and just after birth. If the ewe is stimulated to secrete oxytocin later, she may be persuaded to bond with her lamb then, too. The sense of smell in humans is not as well developed as in animals, but we, too, are more influenced by smell than we imagine.

"I See You"

In higher mammals, and especially in humans, vision also plays an important role during the first meeting with the young. Time and again I have seen babies open their eyes wide at the sight of the tip of a breast. "Hey!" they seem to say. "That exciting round thing I see over there, with a little point at the top, is what I have to get to. Help me, then! Can't you see it's not so easy?"

Early in fetal life, human eyes are sealed shut, just like a newborn kitten's eyes. By birth, though, the baby has been able to see for a long time. When strong sunlight shines on the mother's belly, a beautiful rosy light glows inside the womb, although it is muted, diffuse, not suitable for seeing clearly. Then, all of a sudden, the infant is out in a brightly lit world, with strong daylight, powerful lamps, and lights shining into the baby's eyes.

Putting silver nitrate drops in a baby's eyes to prevent gonorrheal infection was once routine. Like much else, this practice was done with the best of intentions, but with unintended consequences. The first time I worked in a labor ward, I found it difficult to answer the mothers' worried questions about whether these eyedrops were painful for babies. The babies cried, and often their eyes became red and swollen. I reassured the mothers with some trepidation and decided to use myself as a guinea pig to find out. I put the drops in one eye in order to be able to tell the mothers, "No, they hardly notice a thing." I never should have done that. The drops hurt intensely, and my eye became red and so swollen that I could not see anything with it for the rest of the day. I went on rounds with one weeping eye and never again reassured mothers on that point. Instead, I joined the crusade to stop the routine use of silver nitrate eyedrops.

Most newborns today open their eyes and see. Their gaze is incredibly appealing: "Mom! Look at me!" The baby can follow you with that gaze and seems to focus. Research has shown that babies prefer to view a face with shining, open eyes. We don't know enough about what happens during the first eye contact, but it is hardly inconsequential. The practice of goslings is thought-provoking: the young birds follow the first thing that moves in their line of vision—even if it is a wind-up toy or a farmer's boot—and believe it to be their mother forever after.

"It's Cold Out Here!"

The newborn baby gets a bit of a temperature shock after birth. The uterus keeps a constant temperature of 98.6°F, protecting the fetus well against outside influences. It is never colder than this. Then the infant is pushed out to a room temperature of around 68°F; the fact that the baby is all wet makes the air feel even chillier. Newborn babies tolerate temperature loss poorly. They lose warmth in particular from their moist, disproportionately large heads.

French physicians Michel Odent and Frederic Leboyer deserve much credit for the current gentler reception of the newborn, at least where sound, light, and temperature are concerned. Odent and Leboyer advise darkening the room and keeping noise levels low. Their beautiful photos of babies obviously enjoying a dip in warm water are now familiar around the world. The water probably reminds the baby of amniotic fluid; it is reasonable that this is a soothing experience. The baby has the same contented expression when calming down in contact with the mother's body. Today we believe that close, skin-to-skin contact with the mother is even better than warm water for making the transition to life outside as gentle as possible. The baby can have a bath later.

Water Birth

Some people believe that birth should take place in water. A warm bath may relieve pain in the first stage of labor, and labor sometimes progresses so rapidly that the baby is born in the tub. Such a birth usually turns out well. But humans are air-breathing creatures, made for life on land. Granted, the baby has practiced breathing water in and out for months, but during all that time, oxygen has been available through the placenta.

If you run a film of a baby's birth in slow motion, you can see that the chest is compressed as the infant slides out the birth canal, and a stream of fluid comes from the baby's mouth. Outside the mother's body, the baby's chest expands, drawing air into the lungs for the first time. This action is prerequisite for the first cry, and that is how it is meant to work. The lungs are to unfold and start breathing air before the placenta stops sending oxygen to the baby. If the birth happens in a tub, the airways could conceivably be filled instead with contaminated bathwater. Studies have demonstrated, nevertheless, that being born underwater usually works well for the baby, who waits to surface before drawing a first breath. As for the mother, giving birth in water allows her to move about freely, and many women find this less painful.

"Don't Cut My Lifeline Too Soon!"

As long as the umbilical cord is pulsating, there is no rush to do anything. The baby is still getting oxygen from the mother and is also receiving the final blood transfusion from the placenta. In most cases, the child will have a higher hemoglobin level if the cord is cut after pulsation has stopped. On rare occasions, if the mother has antibodies against the baby's blood because of incompatible blood types, the baby may not benefit from this extra blood. In such a case, the cord is cut immediately.

Mammals are generally born downward. The young remain below the level of the uterus and have plenty of time to start breathing before the Wharton's jelly in the umbilical cord expands and stops circulation in it. So why this unnecessary haste in the case of the human infant? Perhaps the baby really is trying hard to say, "Mom and Dad, help me so I can stay anchored as long as it benefits me! It is hard to sort out breathing for someone who's never done it before."

Until birth, babies feel only water at body temperature and the silken membranes of the bag of waters against their skin. After birth, they are dried energetically, with rough towels, to remove blood and amniotic fluid and to stimulate them to take hold and breathe. They are lifted and handled and feel the relative chill, but they also meet warm skin for the first time. All these sensations probably leave strong impressions.

"Are My Exact Weight and Length So Important?"

Necessary stimulation to the newborn is a positive thing. Being removed from mother's warm skin and put on a hard, cold scale, however, will bring out terror in most babies. Stretching the baby to full length in order to obtain a measurement is not an urgent matter. Let the newborn straighten out gradually, without assistance. After all, the infant has just spent many months curved forward. Perhaps the baby can breathe more easily without lying flat on the stomach. Recent research on crib death seems to imply this. Everyone asks about weight and length at once, immediately after learning the baby's gender. Should we change our priorities a bit and concentrate instead on the miracle at hand?

Bathing does not occur on the first day of life in all places, but far too commonly the baby is still washed shortly after birth in water with soap or even in disinfectant—and not rinsed off afterward. What if the baby were to protest? "Here I come, covered with lovely vernix, which protected my skin from being waterlogged by amniotic fluid. It is good for me to keep this natural skin cream. It keeps my skin soft and strong. Don't wash away all the bacteria my mother just gave me. Don't make me fair game for all the hospital bacteria."

Well-meaning people still interfere to bathe and weigh a newborn just as that newborn is working on a great project: bonding with mother and finding the breast. Perhaps it would be better to dip the baby in warm water immediately after birth. Rinsing off blood and other mess is nice before laying the baby on mother's body for a long, undisturbed, get-acquainted session. Drying the baby with warm towels is usually more than sufficient.

Gravity is another surprise for the baby, who was almost weightless when submerged in water. In the womb, the baby became very clever at getting hand to mouth. Many fetuses suck their fingers. Out in the air, the arm suddenly weighs a ton, and familiar movements are slow and unsure.

No wonder, then, that the baby produces significant amounts of the stress hormone adrenaline. No wonder that newborns often have dilated pupils, as we all do when we are afraid or angry. But the baby doesn't seem fearful once calmed down. Instead, the look is one of contemplation and mystery. I often have a diffuse feeling of looking into something unknown through the eyes of a new baby. Is it a greeting from the world the baby has just left behind? "A tiny piece of heaven," said one father.

Other hormones, endorphins, are produced during labor and probably keep the baby from seeming even more horrified over all these changes. Endorphins are the much-discussed "pleasure hormones" that we all experience at times. Because of endorphins, pain is not experienced in the usual way during arousal, whether during somewhat rough love play—or when a soldier is injured in the heat of battle. A baby born vaginally has high endorphin levels. These endorphins probably make the labor less painful for the baby than it would otherwise be. Even babies pulled out by vacuum or forceps seem quite unperturbed after a while.

"Suddenly I Was Just Hauled Out"

But what about the baby born by a planned cesarean section? This baby misses out on a lot. This baby gets no gradual messages about what is about to happen and has no chance to prepare by increasing hormone levels. The lungs of this baby aren't squeezed empty of fluid. Baby apes born by cesarean section are less active and react more slowly than do apes born normally. Human babies born by cesarean section have more problems with beginner's breathing than do babies born vaginally, even when the operation has been performed because of the mother's condition and when the baby itself is completely healthy.

We must do what we can to help babies delivered by cesarean section get the best possible start in life. Mothers whose labors have deviated from the norm in some way often have more problems relating to their babies in the beginning. This may be in part because these mothers miss out on the golden moments of the physical attachment process right after birth, when oxytocin is at its peak. But more opportunities are to come. During any skin-to-skin contact, both mother and baby secrete vital hormones. And every time the baby suckles, the mother secretes oxytocin. This promotes good feelings in her and also helps the baby. Whenever the baby suckles and gets a few drops of milk into the stomach, systems are activated to ensure that the baby gets the mother's scent and appearance stored in memory.

A newborn baby is an intense little creature. Instinctively, the baby has one goal: to reach the breast in order to find food. Many babies need time. Researchers have found, in fact, that the baby's suckling efforts are at maximum strength about ninety minutes after birth. When the baby finally achieves this goal and is lying at the breast experiencing bliss, its feelings are probably something along the lines of, "Hmmm. Maybe life out here isn't so bad after all. I've never tasted anything as good as these drops of colostrum before. Never felt anything so exciting in my mouth as this firm nipple. And never smelled anything as delicious as this soft, brownish skin my nose is resting against. Now I'm safe! Soon I can relax completely and take a good, long nap."

Be aware that the newborn baby:

- Dislikes loud noises and glaring lights.

- Uses vision, hearing, and smell to get acquainted.

- Needs calm, skin contact, and the breast more than bathing, weighing, and measuring.

- Enjoys being touched and spoken to.

CHAPTER 3

Starting Breastfeeding: Like a Duckling to Water?

Did you get off to a golden start, your newborn child in peace at your breast after birth, suckling intensely? If you did, breastfeeding is likely to continue easily and smoothly.

But not everyone gets off to an ideal start, and problems can occur along the way in any case. The baby doesn't always take to the breast like a duckling to water, so here is some further advice to help you on your way.

It has been suggested that the best advice for breastfeeding is to pretend you have been stranded on a deserted island. Both you and your baby are naked. Why? Well, if you were on a deserted island, alone, what would you do each time your baby cried? You would try using the only thing you had readily available to comfort the newborn: you would offer your breast. And because you were both naked, you would hold the smooth little baby very close.

There would be no blankets, diapers, or clothes between you. You would carry the baby on your body all the time. The infant would be constantly stimulated by the skin-to-skin contact and your movements. Often the baby would wake up and demand food, stimulating your breasts into producing a lot of milk. And if your breasts became uncomfortably full, you would probably wake the baby up to suckle and lighten the pressure. The two of you would achieve perfect self-regulation all by yourselves.

LATCHING ON

Remember to let the baby search a little with the mouth before really getting hold of the breast. When the nipple touches the baby's lips, the baby's head starts to wave around and the mouth at the same time opens wider and wider. This is the rooting reflex. Only when the mouth is wide open do you pull the baby in closely against you. This way the mouth is filled with breast as the baby latches on, so that the gnawing is not just on the nipple, which would make the nipple sore. Milking is easier when the baby has a large hold; after all, the process is called "breastfeeding," not "nipplefeeding." The first few sucks on an engorged breast can be a bit uncomfortable, but breastfeeding should otherwise not hurt.

No Pulling on the Nipple

Draw the baby very close, perhaps with your hand on the back of the baby's shoulders. This keeps the baby from "hanging" from the breast, which pulls on the nipple and can overstretch it, leading to cracks around the base.

The Baby's Chin against Your Breast

When you hold your baby close, leaving the head free, the tiny chin will automatically be pressed against your breast. This is especially good for expressing milk. In addition, it makes the baby's head bend back a little so that the nose comes just free of the breast and the baby breathes through a tiny gap. Unless your breast is very large and soft, you should not have to push on it to keep it away from the baby's nose.

You Should Enjoy Breastfeeding, too

Before you left the maternity ward, did anyone show you how to breastfeed both sitting up and lying down? You will need to be able to breastfeed both ways. When your baby is lying snugly against you and has a nice latch-on, check whether you are comfortable yourself. Tense muscles will leave you exhausted, instead of relaxed and rested, when the baby is finished feeding.

It is better to feed lying down when you need a rest, when you are almost asleep, or if you have painful stitches after giving birth. Lie with one shoulder directly on the mattress and put plenty of pillows under your head. Check that your head is supported so that you can see your baby without lifting your head or tensing up.

You have to lie with your body in a stable sideways position to avoid tipping over. Perhaps drawing one knee up will stabilize you. Feel that your arms are resting even when you are holding your baby. To get some additional support, wrap a blanket or comforter closely around you both; with this done, you won't have to make an effort to hold your baby close enough, and your baby will keep a good suckling hold and won't fall out of bed even if you fall asleep.

BREASTFEEDING WHILE SEATED

If your arms are not supported, the baby you hold will get very heavy. With experience, many women end up in a position often seen in primitive societies, sitting low and leaning forward slightly, supporting their arms on their thighs or with one knee laid over the other. Some use a little footstool to get their thighs higher up while sitting in a chair.

Particularly in the beginning, it is important that you be conscious of the need to support your arms, either on the armrests of your chair, on a special nursing cushion, or with some other firm support. Otherwise, as soon as your baby has been lifted, latched onto your breast, and gotten a good suckling hold, your arms will gradually become tired and inevitably sink down. As a consequence, your baby ends up hanging from your nipple, pulling on it and making it sore, often causing cracking around the base. Check to make sure that you are sitting with your shoulders lowered and your arms relaxed. Make sure that you don't tense up between the shoulder blades and that the rest of your back is comfortable.

HOW OFTEN DO YOU NURSE?

You should offer the breast every time your baby shows interest in it. Remember that this same infant was nourished continuously in the womb. Getting used to spacing meals takes time. Breast milk is very easy to digest and passes quickly through the stomach.

After about a week, most babies want approximately twelve meals over a twenty-four-hour period. Many of them later want less frequent feeding, but others keep demanding food at short intervals for many months. Simply offering the breast is usually less strenuous than trying to comfort the baby in other ways.

If you keep your baby around you all the time, you will quickly learn to read the signals of hunger before any upset leads to crying. Recognizing the signals and responding early will make it easier for the baby to latch on well to your breast.

How Long Do You Nurse?

Within reasonable limits, it is a good idea to let your baby decide how long to nurse. Even before your breasts are producing much milk, it is important that the baby gets to suckle a lot. This gives strong signals to your body that a hungry newborn baby needs food. Nearly all breasts respond willingly to sufficient signals.

To begin, the baby must suckle long enough for the signals to reach the pituitary gland in your brain. This is where the hormone oxytocin is produced. Only when this hormone is released into the blood and reaches the breast will the tiny bundles of muscle around the milk stores contract so that the milk is squeezed out. After a while, the milk will drip or even spray out automatically when this letdown reflex starts working. This was one of the tragic things about the breastfeeding failures a few decades ago: just as the letdown reflex was about to set in, the baby was removed from the breast when someone came and said, "Only five minutes the first few days . . ."

The amount of prolactin, the hormone that controls the amount of milk, also increases strongly during breastfeeding. If suckling is interrupted after ten minutes, the level of prolactin is only a fraction of what it would be if the baby were left to suckle for half an hour. The motto for developing a sufficient amount of milk is almost biblical: the more you give, the more you shall receive!

If you are aware of these simple things, breastfeeding is not likely to pose any problems for you. It often takes a little time before everything works smoothly, however. Breastfeeding can be compared to making love. If neither of the partners is experienced, the couple is bound to be a little clumsy at first. If one partner has some experience, it works better. When both have learned what it's all about, they usually get along just fine.

If you are finding breastfeeding a strain, perhaps you will recognize one of the problems in the following pages and find some useful advice.

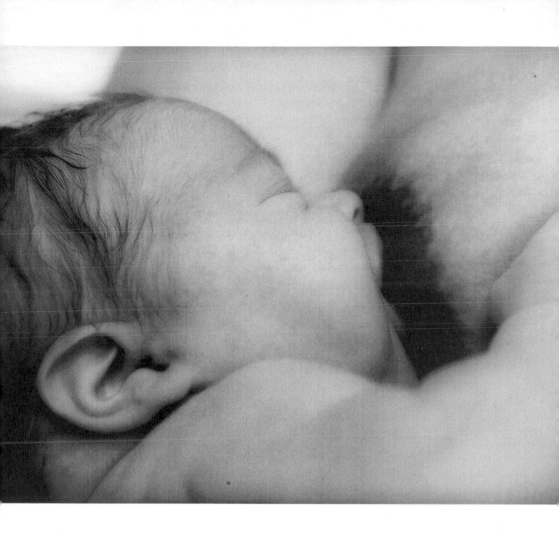

The Baby Doesn't Latch onto the Breast Properly

Failure of the baby to latch on properly is one of the most frequent breastfeeding problems in the maternity ward. We often suspect that the baby has been a bit sedated by the pain-relief medication that the mother may have received during labor.

Sometimes the shape of the nipple—which can be quite large or flat or not very stretchable—can cause problems. Perhaps you have given birth to a baby with a little rosebud mouth instead of the large gullet that most newborns present. Perhaps you have both problems.

In these cases, you need help from someone with experience. You must work to get your baby to search and open the mouth wide and do the other things described earlier. The nipple must be stimulated to become erect and easier for the baby to get hold of. If the baby's mouth doesn't make this happen, you can help out with a few clean fingers. This may all seem hopeless for a few days, but try to remember that a small mouth grows quickly. In addition, the sedating medication eventually leaves the baby's body; much of it is gone after a few days (although weeklong aftereffects have been reported). Some babies may need to be given breast milk by cup or spoon for a short period while they practice at the breast.

Sometimes the problem is a hard, swollen, perhaps engorged breast; the baby can't get a good suckling hold and just nibbles the nipple. Little milk comes out, and the baby ends up damaging the delicate skin. The solution in this case is to let out a little milk so that the dark area around the nipple—the areola—becomes soft and stretchable again and can form a good long "nipple." Hand-milking is often the gentlest way to do this.

If you allow your baby to suckle often, your breasts quickly learn how much milk is needed and do not become overfull or engorged. If your baby starts sleeping through the night quite early, this might prove a dubious advantage. You may get a longer period of unbroken sleep but then wake up to face breastfeeding problems.

THE BABY TAKES SMALL AMOUNTS OF MILK AND LOSES A LOT OF WEIGHT

The milk of first-time mothers usually really sets in after about three days; this happens a little earlier for those who have given birth before. In general, the earlier suckling starts—and the more the baby is allowed to feed after birth—the more quickly the milk comes. But all women are made differently. Some have milk even before the baby is born, while others have to wait longer. Don't forget that babies born at term have a store of sugar in their livers to help them survive until the milk really sets in.

The most common reason for milk not to start flowing as expected is that stimulation of the breast is insufficient. This may be because sucking is weak or because suckling time is too short.

Perhaps you have given birth to a modest little person who lies nibbling politely at your breast? In former times, when fear of dangerous infections was less, a mother who didn't have enough milk might borrow a strong-sucking baby from another mother a few times. Nursing that baby could help her breasts to get the signal and increase milk production.

There are ways to stimulate sucking. One is to unwrap and allow your baby to cool down a little. Research has shown that this may make the sucking more energetic. Another is to firmly massage the baby's palms and soles of the feet to stimulate the gripping reflex, the same reflex that allows our relatives the ape babies to cling to their mother's fur. The gripping reflex in turn stimulates the sucking reflex.

Perhaps the baby has a passing period of weaker sucking because of jaundice and a need for phototherapy. This stressful situation brings many tears from new mothers. The yellow color of jaundice is caused by the pigment that forms with the breaking down of many fetal blood cells that the baby no longer needs. Light treatment helps this process. At such a time, the baby benefits from sucking a lot. The more she eats, the more bowel movements are stimulated. Each time the baby passes stool, some of the yellow bilirubin also passes out. If the bilirubin stays too long in the gut, it may be reabsorbed and have to go through the body again.

Jaundiced babies need food, and mother's milk is the very best. Take the baby out of the light to nurse every few hours. If you have plenty of milk, there is no reason to give the baby any other nourishment or fluids. If your milk hasn't really set in yet, the baby may need supplementary feedings for a short while. But always offer the breast first!

You can help a placid baby by gripping both cheeks to force a pout during feeding. Massage both cheeks a little; massaging just one cheek usually makes the baby turn toward that side and lose the suckling hold. Some babies get an extra stimulus to their nervous system by lying with their body under the mother's arm, legs bent at the knee and hip joints and soles of the feet propped against a firm surface. But first and last, check the suckling hold. Only a lot of soft breast in the baby's mouth will stimulate all the way up the palate, which is where the real sucking reflex is elicited.

The maternity period is stressful. A lot of things happen at once. Your body has to adjust after giving birth; you have to learn a lot; you have to care for yourself and your baby; receive visitors; and so on. Perhaps enough time has not been left for breastfeeding. The best remedy for this situation is to take "feed and rest" days. Many good maternity wards have a system for this. If the baby is losing a lot of weight or seems dissatisfied, the mother is told to spend as much time as possible resting in bed. She should have food brought to her, someone else to change her baby, something good to drink. Some people suggest a sip of non-alcoholic beer; others prefer special teas. Beer has actually been shown to have a positive effect on milk production. The mother should receive only short visits. The one thing only she can do is breastfeed—and she should do it a lot. A baby who doesn't wake up wanting food should be carefully roused, preferably every other hour during the day and several times at night. Suckling must be allowed to continue until the baby lets go. The mother should also try to take several naps throughout the day. After a day or two of this intensive breastfeeding and rest, most mothers will wake up with plenty of milk, and the baby will put on weight nicely.

A Delayed Letdown Reflex

After a few days, if you can't hear your baby swallowing after a little while at the breast, the letdown reflex might not be working properly yet. Try to stimulate the other breast while the baby is suckling. Rub that breast, massage it, roll the nipple, anything. Such stimulation increases the hormone level (even when you are not feeding) and eases the letdown. All skin contact increases the oxytocin level. In addition to generally helping with relaxation and well-being, touch is beneficial for breastfeeding. In some cultures, a nursing mother receives a daily massage. This stimulates extra waves of oxytocin, which reduce a worried mother's anxieties and probably also make her milk flow more easily. A mother might also benefit from getting a massage. If you are on your own, try caring for yourself by using a mild moisturizing lotion before breastfeeding or by cuddling skin-to-skin with your baby.

If your baby suckles for only a short time, give your breasts a little extra stimulation between feedings, even on the outside of your clothes, while you relax and do other things. Dad can also be a very willing assistant.

Sore Nipples

Breastfeeding should never hurt. The breasts often do feel tender, however, especially in the beginning, when the baby takes the first strong sucks on an unprepared or very full breast. After a short while, when the pressure eases off and the breast softens, breastfeeding should not be uncomfortable, but rather to the contrary. The fat hindmilk left on the nipple after feeding normally provides all the care the nipple needs. Just let it dry in the air. Do not manipulate the nipple unless your fingers are completely clean.

The nipple will often be sore at the tip if the baby has been gnawing it or rubbing it with the tongue. If the baby has been pulling, the nipple may have cracks around the base. If the nipple is deformed and crooked when it leaves the baby's mouth, it has been subjected to uneven pressure. Play detective and try to find out what isn't working well.

You can often find an alternative position for the baby to avoid putting pressure on the sore area. For example, the baby can "stand up" while nursing. Standing can also be a good nursing position for a baby with a blocked nose. Alternatively, the mother can tuck the baby under her arm.

If you are already sore, many tips and remedies and all kinds of creams and ointments are available to you. Unless the problem that led to the soreness is solved, however, none of these things will do you much good. You can spare the sorer breast by starting nursing on the better one and then moving the baby over when the milk has started running. Or you can start the letdown reflex by stimulating the nipple a little before you put the baby to the breast.

If the baby's suckling hold and closeness to your body are correct but you still have a sore or a crack that won't heal, a little ointment on just that one spot can help. The main rule for treating sores is to keep dry and use wet on wet. This means that you should allow the sound, unaffected skin to air-dry, keeping it as dry as possible until the next feeding. The moist sore will heal more quickly and less painfully, however, if you cover it with a little salve or a compress moistened with saline solution. A tube of salve with a small, pointed end can make application easy.

One strong warning against breast creams in general is that you should not apply them to the entire nipple and areola immediately after feeding; doing so leaves the healthy skin damp under the cream and does not allow it to dry as it should. Applying creams in this way is similar to wearing a rubber glove on a wet hand: the skin stays moist and becomes vulnerable and nonresistant. If the nipples feel rough like chapped lips despite being left to air-dry, you can, of course, put a small amount of mild cream on them.

Remember that the bumps on the areola are oil glands, which are supposed to protect against the moistness of breastfeeding. Don't wash this oil away with soap. Also remember that covering the breast with artificial emollients all the time may reduce production of the breast's own very best protecting agents.

The breast also becomes vulnerable if wrapped in damp nursing pads or a milk-sodden bra. In addition, the bra presses the nipple inward, where it remains moist, skin against skin, instead of drying freely. Leave your chest bare whenever possible! If your breasts are heavy, let them rest on top of a bra, or open the flaps of a nursing bra. If the maternity ward has a lot of visitors, leave your chest bare under a loose shirt and change your shirt when you need to. A little sunshine can also be good.

Rounded cups placed inside the bra to gather dripping milk allow the nipples to "come out" and stand free rather than to be squeezed flat by a bra. Cups with a perforated upper part and a large opening for the areola and nipple are the most comfortable. You can find these cups at a pharmacy. When you use such a cup, the nipple is free and dry, poking out into the air. If resorting to such devices feels uncomfortable, remember that the nipple was not originally meant to be damp and flattened by clothing. Some people find the most comfortable thing is simply to cut a small hole in the bra for the nipple.

Nursing pads or the fabric of a bra can stick to sore skin. When the pad or fabric is removed, the scab often follows, along with the new skin forming underneath. This prevents healing and should be avoided. Anything stuck to a sore nipple should be thoroughly soaked with clean water until it can be removed without causing damage. If sore nipples do not heal even after you have followed all of this advice, have a bacterial swab taken. Often an infection is sustaining such soreness and needs treatment.

Breast shields placed between the baby's mouth and the breast during breastfeeding are rarely useful, although there are exceptions. If the nipple remains very flat in spite of proper stimulation and it is difficult for the baby to get hold of a large mouthful of breast, the nipple of such a shield may make it easier for the baby to latch on. Also, very rarely the mothers nipples may be so sore that she can't stand for the baby to suck directly on her breast. But usually using a shield should be a last resort and is only a short-term solution. The baby may take less milk when a breast shield is used, even with the thin silicone shields shaped to fit the nipple. This is because the breasts are not stimulated well through the shield. Whether the baby isn't sucking well or the breast is sore, shields don't solve the underlying problem.

During a problem-solving session in a maternity ward, several nurses were quite enthusiastic about breast shields, because they felt that breast shields could solve some difficult problems. Angela was described as an example. She had used breast shields with her first two children and had asked for them this time as well. She had just gone home with her exclusively breastfed baby, with breast shields. This sounded good, and the nursing staff clearly felt confident that she would be problem free.

Two days later, Angela called. When I examined her, she had all the symptoms of mastitis. One of her nipples was sore, and she had used a shield every time she breastfed on that side. It turned out that she had given up breastfeeding relatively early with her first two children because she hadn't had enough milk. The maternity ward had known nothing about this. This last time, she had indeed breastfed exclusively—mainly from her one good breast. The other breast, with the shield, had also been suckled frequently, but it had not been properly emptied, which had resulted in high fever and a swollen, red, painful breast. After Angela expressed a little milk by hand, she helped her baby find his own way. He latched on nicely without the shield and emptied her breast quite well. Angela and her husband were shown how to help their son get a good suckling hold and were reminded of the importance of proper emptying. Twenty-four hours later, the mastitis and the breast shield were both distant memories.

It is often difficult to wean a baby off a breast shield. Always offer the breast first, soft and pliable and without the shield, to a not-too-hungry baby. If that doesn't work, gradually—day by day—snip a little more off the nipple of the shield until only the surrounding ring is left; then, finally, remove that as well.

TWINS

Advice for breastfeeding twins is mainly the same as advice for breast-feeding only one child. You usually have to expect some extra-busy weeks to start with twins, however. In the beginning, when both mother and babies are practicing, most women feed one child at a time. If the twins are good suckers and get to the breast often enough, milk production will increase to meet demand. Most women can make enough milk for two babies.

There is no simpler and cheaper way to feed twins than by exclusive breastfeeding. Although this usually means frequent feeding, it ultimately saves time as well. If possible, a mother of twins should let someone else do all the housework and child care. After a while, try feeding the twins simultaneously. You may decide that you prefer to feed one baby at a time, but you should nonetheless learn how to feed both together, a skill that will be handy if both are hungry at the same time or if you are in a hurry.

Animals are practical in this way. A sheep will let each lamb suckle at any time for the first few weeks, but after a while, the hungry lamb must bring along its twin before any milk is to be had. The same goes for a sow, who signals to all her piglets when it's feeding time. Only when all are in place does she let down her milk, accompanied by a new tone in her grunting.

Many mothers of twins find a special nursing cushion very useful, while others build up a cushion support in the bed or on the sofa. The babies can be placed with their bodies across each other or with one body under each of the mother's arms, or they can be angled the same way. While the mother is on her back, she may have one baby on either side, propped up by pillows. Some twins choose a favorite breast each. Disadvantages to this could be that their eyes always look up at the same angle during feeding and that they get somewhat one-sided stimulation.

Mothers who give birth to more than two children at the same time usually try to give some breast milk to each baby, even if it is only a portion of each baby's food. Two women who have given birth to triplets at the National Hospital in Oslo in recent years contacted me afterward and told me that they had fed all three on their own milk for months, but these women are likely exceptions. Triplets and quadruplets are most often premature and greatly need the advantages of breast milk. These mothers must decide when they have had enough, however—the work of breastfeeding or pumping and using supplements in addition to everything else can be exhausting. Although breastfeeding is generally the ideal, given the variables and complications associated with multiple births, formula may be a good alternative for these babies and can help them grow well, too.

To start breastfeeding successfully:

- Let your baby sniff, search, open the mouth wide, and take a lot of breast in the mouth.

- Make sure your baby has a large latch-on.

- Make sure that your baby's lower lip is curled outward.

- Check that your baby's chin is close against your breast.

- Express some milk from a hard breast if your baby cannot get a proper hold.

- Hold your baby close, facing you.

- Sit or lie comfortably—without tense muscles.

- Let your baby suckle often enough—at least twelve times in twenty-four hours, preferably more.

- Let suckling continue for long enough—usually until the baby lets go.

- Wake a baby who sleeps too long between feedings during the day and does not gain enough weight.

WHAT TO EXPECT FROM A HOSPITAL THAT SUPPORTS BREASTFEEDING

Before you give birth, you will be informed of the advantages of breast milk and the best way to get started with breastfeeding so that you are well prepared.

Immediately after giving birth, you will be given your baby to keep undisturbed, skin-to-skin, for at least one hour or until the first breastfeeding has taken place. This is to give your baby an opportunity to go through the stages of searching and succeeding at the breast.

If the first breastfeeding has to be postponed because of a cesarean section or other complications, you will be given your baby within half an hour after you make a request and are able to relate to your baby.

Healthcare staff will check from the beginning to make sure that everything is going well with your breastfeeding. You will receive guidance when you need it, as often as you need it. If problems arise, you will receive help to solve them.

If you are temporarily separated from your baby, you will be shown how to express milk manually and how to use a breast pump, and you will learn what is needed to maintain milk production.

If your baby has to stay in the pediatric ward, you will be able to stay there too for most of the day if you want to.

Your newborn baby will not receive any form of nutrition or fluid other than breast milk unless there is a medical reason for giving it.

During your stay in the maternity ward, you will be able to keep your baby with you around the clock if you want to. You will also be offered a break from it if you are tired. The staff will care for you so that you can save your strength for your baby.

You will be encouraged to breastfeed on demand. This means that your baby may suck as soon as interest is shown and for as long as the baby wants, within reasonable limits, if this is OK with you.

You will learn that very sleepy babies who do not demand to be fed should be picked up, carried, and stimulated and that you can waken a baby and put the baby to your breast if you want to—if your breasts are very full, for example.

A pacifier or bottle will not be used in the maternity ward. You will be advised to avoid these things until breastfeeding is well established and you have plentiful and stable milk production.

You will receive information about where you can get help if breastfeeding problems arise. You will be informed about La Leche League groups and how you can join one. These requirements conform with the ten steps for successful breastfeeding specified by UNICEF and the World Health Organization.

. . .

CHAPTER 4

Dad in the Postpartum Period

DEAR NEW DAD

Even if much revolves around your baby's mother right now, you are equally important—just in a different way. Without you, there would be no baby. Half of the baby has grown from your genetic material. When the one selected sperm from among your millions wiggled its way to the egg, this special baby of yours was formed, unique in the world.

Whether or not a baby was wanted at the outset, there is a big chance that you, as a modern man, have also participated actively since the fertilization. You have probably sat with your hand on your partner's stomach and felt small kicks. Chances are you have lain with your ear pressed against her skin and listened for the fetal heart. You were most likely there during the ultrasound examination, the pregnancy, the birth.

Perhaps you think that this is the greatest thing you have ever experienced, that the birth itself was a miracle. Perhaps you have forged an even closer bond to your partner, who has given birth to your baby. Or perhaps a part of you—secretly—is slightly disappointed or even repulsed?

A DIFFICULT BIRTH

Mark, who was twenty-eight when his first baby was born, said he felt afterward that there was so little he could do and that what he did do didn't help much. The birth was more violent than he had imagined, more animal-like. He was uncommonly frank and mentioned the smells: blood, sex, amniotic fluid, sweat, urine, feces. He talked of the noises: moans and cries that he had thought belonged to passionate lovemaking. These sounds made him rather embarrassed to look at the birth attendants, and he wondered whether they thought the same. Yet sex had never seemed more distant than when he had seen Mona's unrecognizable genitals right after the birth. She was split and bleeding and had to have a lot of stitches. He felt sick and had to concentrate hard on the baby and on looking enthusiastic in the middle of all the chaos. He constantly had the feeling of playing second fiddle. It had been like that all through the pregnancy as well, but during the birth, especially, it was all about Mona, poor thing. And when the baby finally appeared, Mark even had to play third fiddle. Everything revolved around the mother and baby, mother and baby.

THE BIG PROTECTOR

Mark was surprised when strong protective feelings suddenly flared up inside him. He smiled at it afterward. "I thought that I'd be in seventh heaven when everything was finally over and the baby lay at the breast and we were surrounded by peace and quiet. But I became awfully irritable. I thought that they didn't look after Mona properly, that there was too much fuss with the baby. After all, it was ours. I wanted to rush at the nurse who had been so great earlier, when she came and checked the baby for the nth time. I just wanted to position myself in front of Mona and the baby, to shield them. Actually, I was ready to fight for them. I think I hid it quite well, but I wanted everyone else to get lost. This was actually one of the reasons why I sent a big box of chocolates to the department afterward. Inside, I felt that I had been ungrateful even though I managed to hide it pretty well."

Such feelings are actually OK, because they probably express care. And care and responsibility are exactly what are needed from a father from the start. You should be the one to look after and make arrangements for the baby's fumbling start, which should mainly take place with the mother. You have had a strong experience. But it is her body that has labored, suffered, and conquered. In addition, her hormones will fluctuate wildly in the hours after birth. They affect both her emotions and the way she behaves. No one benefits from your trying to act as much like her as possible at this time. You have your own independent masculine role. The best thing for all three of you is for you to keep a foothold and a lookout. You can contribute to obtaining peace and

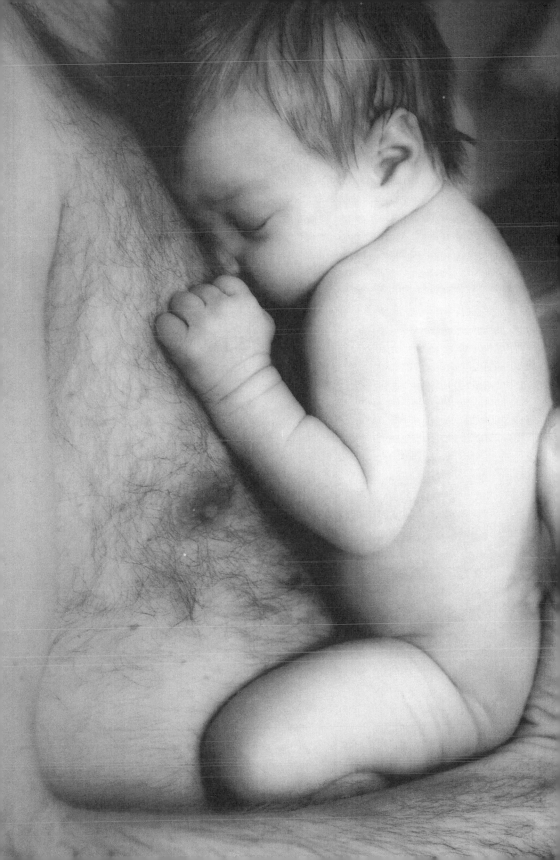

quiet, or you can get help when it is needed. It is only right that the two of you are different.

Just after the birth, the woman may seem to need the man to recognize the baby, to show that he accepts the baby as his own. One of the most common exclamations from women who have just given birth is, "I think he looks like you." Perhaps this is to bond the man to the baby?

It is also important that the father recognize his partner's performance—not like one new father, who said, "Are you sure that you did it right? You didn't seem to be pushing the way you were taught in Lamaze class." Remember: irrespective of how it all went, she has delivered the performance of her life.

A Good Second

You are temporarily a good second in relation to the baby. But your time will come, and it will come faster and more intensely than you realize. It is probably good if you also touch the baby a bit in the hours after birth. The baby, normally born sterile, is now about to be colonized, or infected with bacteria. Most of these bacteria are harmless, but some may cause illness. It is beneficial if the mother is the first to transfer her own bacteria to the baby—not the hospital staff, who often have a different and less favorable bacterial flora. After the mother, I believe that the father is best, because he and the mother have many bacteria in common. They share a bed, kiss, make love, often eat the same things, are exposed to the same infectious diseases, and so on. Many of the antibodies in the breast milk also provide protection against the father's bacteria.

One Native American tribe has an expression for the parents' roles in relation to a new baby. It goes roughly like this: "The mother should give the baby confidence in the world; the father should teach the baby to conquer it." And you certainly will do that! You will teach your baby to swim, to draw, to cope with life. But now, when your baby is completely new, is there anything you can do? Of course there is! You can increasingly hold that baby, caress her, look after him. Be aware, though, that some women become uneasy when other people handle their baby at the outset. You may feel hurt if this includes you. This may be related to the vigilance of animal mothers against letting anyone come near their newborn offspring. Perhaps instinct controls this in part, and perhaps this vigilance should be respected completely in the very beginning. Having a new baby is tough, and a lot necessarily falls to a breastfeeding mother. It is important that she get help from all possible instincts, reflexes, and hormones.

What Can We Learn from Other Species?

Jane Goodall, who has done fieldwork among chimpanzees in Africa for more than thirty years, describes what typically happens when a new youngster is born. The mother isolates herself with her baby for a while. Then the other female chimpanzees gather around the mother and baby and watch keenly, while the adult males keep well away. Other than the mother, the first to touch the baby are usually older siblings. An older sister is eventually allowed to tend to the young one. According to an interesting description of big apes in captivity, the grandmother and aunts are once in a while allowed to tend to even quite a small infant. The few times a male shows interest in the infant, the mother is uneasy and tense. Humans are not apes, and apes do not live as male-female couples. Nevertheless, it is interesting to look to the apes when we try to understand our behavior regarding newborn babies.

Yellow baboon mothers are apt to find a male baboon, often the youngster's father, to protect them. He feeds the infant small morsels of adult food and even lets it ride on his back. Most important, he protects the mother so that she can find food and look after the little one undisturbed.

Mammals are unique in that their offspring, in addition to growing inside the mother, are also fed by her for a long period. All female mammals, including humans, have a similar hormone pattern during pregnancy, birth, and breastfeeding. This pattern contributes to the fact that the mother is normally intensely preoccupied with her offspring and feeds and protects it. The male, in contrast, shows varying behavior. It is difficult to know whether any pattern is inborn in the human father. Apparently he has countless possible reactions, depending on which culture he has grown up in.

Cats demonstrate an interesting example of the variation in paternal behavior within one species. The male of the cat family is often a real bad guy. A lion, or a tomcat, is apt to kill off any young that are not his own offspring. A built-in need to promote his own genes drives him. After the young grow up and are no longer dependent on the mother, the female is soon ready to mate again.

Female cats often mate with several males, a strategy that makes an adult male less likely to kill her young. If he did, he would risk killing his own offspring. The interesting thing, however, is that cats organize themselves very differently. Actually, researchers have never found two cat societies exactly alike. Some male cats dominate a harem in a specific range. Other cats live in lifelong monogamy. Anyone who has had a couple of house cats become parents has observed how the daddy lovingly participates in the care of the kittens. He licks, warms, and comforts them and defends them when need be, a far cry from the prowling, kitten-murdering tomcat.

ONLY DAD CAN BE DAD

Research shows that men who spend a lot of time with their newborn babies form a stronger emotional bond with them. Also, even the father often makes his voice lighter when he talks to his little one, and he kisses and delights in the baby. Skin-to-skin contact causes the hormone oxytocin to increase in men as well as in women, although at a lower level. In animals, increased care for the offspring correlates with rising levels of oxytocin. Although parents appear to show particular tenderness to babies of the sex opposite their own, the father eventually plays more robustly with his boy baby. Many babies show early on that they find their dad more fun and exciting to be with than their mother. Then it is her turn to feel left out.

Instincts help women and men in different ways, especially with regard to procreation. An interesting experiment demonstrates this. A team of researchers tried to find the most arresting advertising images. Subjects were positioned opposite an apparatus that measured pupil size. (The pupils dilate independently of one's will. Dilation is an instinctive reaction and indicates interest and extra alertness.) The subjects were then shown pictures. A sure way to get a reaction in the pupils of most men was to show them a picture of a naked woman. Pictures of naked men, in contrast, did not provoke a similar reaction in women. Can you guess what made the women's pupils dilate? Correct: the picture of a newborn baby. This is quite simple and clever, really. Instincts, after all, are mostly about the survival of the species, in this case procreation. For a new generation to grow up, the man, strictly speaking, needs only to react to the woman, whereas the woman must react to the baby. Everything else to do with women's pleasure over the male body and with men's love of small children should perhaps be counted as fringe benefits with regard to the preservation of the species.

I do not mean that men are not interested in their newborn offspring. On the contrary, most of them are filled with loving pride. As a completely new dad, however, you do not have the same support from biology as the woman has.

Here is an everyday example: We visited a middle-aged couple who had just become grandparents. The son of the house and his wife came on their first visit with their week-old son. Relatives and friends gathered to congratulate the new parents. The men slapped the father on the back and joked a little but otherwise sat down and talked about their own affairs. The women, in contrast, crowded around the mother and baby, marveled at the little one, and talked baby talk to him with soft, light voices. The women asked the young mother about the birth. They all showed a keen interest and wanted to contribute their own experiences. Problems were discussed and good advice and experiences shared.

By the time the young couple went home after a few hours, all the women had been allowed to hold the baby, although several had held back for a long time before they asked nicely whether they could do so. The new mother, pale and tired, swelled visibly with pride. She looked with renewed interest and love at this crying baby with whom she was actually quite fed up. He had kept her awake all night and was untiring in his demands. Now he was suddenly a privilege again, a treasure that others envied her, that she could share with them.

None of the men had held the baby, and one had even responded with distaste: "Perhaps I shouldn't say this, but I'm a bit scared of these little ones." Yes, perhaps so—and also not very interested so early on?

It was once fairly common to hear men say, "These newborn babies aren't for me. I find them a bit repulsive, and I'm frightened of holding them. It's more fun when they begin to smile, become people . . ." Today, only men who do not have children, or who had them many years ago, say this. Don't modern fathers have such feelings? Or do they dare not express them openly? In any case, certainly their own fathers rarely provided clear role models for them. Today's young dads are the first generation of men to be fully involved in caring for their newborn baby. This is a sociologically interesting development.

Whether you feel ready for this or not, you, the father, may be the first person the baby gets to know outside the womb. This can happen after a cesarean section under full general anesthesia, for example. You should be prepared to give your baby skin contact and to make calming sounds, to make the infant feel safe and confident in this new frightening world, even if contact with the mother will have to wait.

It is also important in the hours after birth that you acknowledge that normally neither you nor other people should disturb the instinctive and hormonal interaction that will bring the baby to the first successful breastfeeding. Too much "fair" sharing just then can create problems in the long term.

It's a Busy Life Being a Dad

Jack wrote to me that he thinks it is important to prepare fathers for how busy the days following the birth will be. He had thought he would have time off for himself while Sally was at the hospital. "No way!" he realized later. "I was mostly at the hospital and was wound up in what was happening there. I spent the rest of the time on the phone, shopping, washing, and tidying up at home. It is important that as much as possible is done before the birth." Some fathers even stay with mother and baby in a family room at the hospital. Even more time is taken up then.

"Me, Jealous?"

It means a lot that you are aware and supportive of the fact that breast milk is best for your baby—and that you contribute as best you can to help the breastfeeding be successful. Sometimes a new father may be a bit envious. It can even happen that a new father says, "It's so sad not to be able to feed the baby. What if I give him a bottle, at night, for example?" On the whole, it is not a good idea to give the baby anything other than breast milk at the beginning, and even that should not be given in a bottle before breastfeeding is well established and the baby has had a lot of experience with sucking on the breast. You can be the one to carry and comfort a baby who cries inconsolably in the night even after breastfeeding, giving the mother a few hours to sleep and then bringing them back together for another breastfeeding.

It is usually most practical for the mother to deal with the baby during the night, however. Most babies need feeding several times, and it seems impractical for the father to get up when the mother is normally also awake at the first whimper and has what is needed. My husband and I had an agreement regarding our youngest child. I would take the night for the first year, and then he would get up and comfort her later on when she woke at night.

One form of jealousy is not necessarily easy to talk about. A friend put it like this: "I have always loved my wife's breasts. I'm quite fixated on boobs. It felt a bit strange when the most sexy part of her was suddenly transformed into feeding stations to which another guy continually had first option. They also leaked every time I fondled them." Evidently this emotion is not so easy to tackle and is slightly embarrassing. Another father, in contrast, might swell in triple delight that his sexuality has led to his baby being fed by his woman. And some women say that their husbands particularly enjoy the fullness, the moistness, and the taste of their dripping breasts.

You may also feel a bit sensitive as a new dad if an experienced woman—the baby's grandmother, for example—is more useful than you are to start with. Many young women need their mother at this time. The Virgin Mary is sometimes shown holding her infant son and sitting on the lap of her mother, Anna. In this portrayal, Mary has the constant support and care of her own big—*grand*—mother.

A One-Man Support System?

Most Norwegian fathers take two weeks' paternity leave when mother and baby come home, and then another four weeks sometime during the first year. This is still uncommon in most of the world. Whatever leave you are entitled to, perhaps you can split up the time. Maybe your constant presence will be more useful and more fun after a few weeks, when mother has recovered slightly, when Granny has returned home (if she ever came), when the breastfeeding has really got going. Think about it. A colleague of mine got permission to delay his paternity leave when his wife gave birth to their fourth child. Six months later, the whole family rented a house in Italy. Be aware, though, that according to the rules (at least in Norway), a father's paternity leave of two weeks is to be taken in connection with the birth.

Whenever a leave is taken, most fathers have to go back to work a while after the birth. This creates a new situation in the couple's relationship. As a childless working couple, you perhaps met for cozy late-night dinners or ate out with friends. Now it is more important that you get home early, that you have a regular schedule. It is not appropriate or right that one adult should be alone for long days with a small baby. If the new mother does not have close contact with other adults during the day, it is suddenly you who has to replace both colleagues and other contact networks. Make time for this. Perhaps she really needs to get away from the baby for a while. In this case, you can take your new child out for a ride in the stroller to give mother an hour completely to herself. More commonly, she will want to do something with other adults, together with you and the baby.

Another job that you have as a new father is to understand and accept her emotions. Perhaps the sensible woman you fell in love with will appear quite different for a while. You think that everything is fine; she is worried and tired. You want to comfort her physically; she wants to be left in peace. You want life to return to normal socially as quickly as possible; she needs to progress gradually. You believe that by now the child should be getting into a rhythm, but this will probably take months. She needs for you to take care of the basics, to sort out the world outside. This may also include managing visits from others to see her and the new baby: "Yes, if you bring the cake—and leave in an hour."

Even if you are feeling a bit sorry for yourself because you can't breastfeed, you can and should help out in other ways at this time. Do the cleaning and the laundry, cook meals, and do the shopping. Bring small surprises home: flowers when the ones she was given at the hospital have withered, some pastry, a ripe avocado, breakfast in bed, a little romantic attention. Your role at the start is to create good conditions for her so that she can give your baby security and milk.

In addition, you can do many things with the baby yourself. Many new fathers gradually discover to their joy that they are even better at comforting the baby than the mother is, especially when the baby cries without being hungry. And from six months on, you can also feed the baby. The father, in fact, often finds it easier to get the baby to accept new food than the mother does, because the mother is associated with breast milk. From now on, you will notice that your importance as a dad steadily increases. The best of luck to you!

Dad, you are especially important when you:

- Make sure that mother and baby are undisturbed, with you, in the hours after the birth.

- Carry and quiet the baby who cries for reasons other than hunger.

- Take care of everything other than the baby and breastfeeding to begin with.

- Make healthy and satisfying meals and drinks for the mother, as she is the one who feeds the baby.

- Encourage the mother by pointing out to her that initial problems are common and worth the effort to surmount.

- Put up with a milk-leaking, bleeding, weepy person for a while.

- Accept that your needs and love life will come after the baby's needs for a while.

- Make sure that a tired mother can sleep when you look after the baby for the odd night and just go to her when the baby needs feeding.

- Gradually start going for walks, diverting, and entertaining the baby.

CHAPTER 5

. . .

Waiting for the Joy of Motherhood

Finally, the birth is over. Now the baby—he or she—has arrived, the little one who has lived inside your body for so long. New, warm emotions bubble up inside you; you are totally in love with your baby. You feel happy. Great, then; you do not need to read any further.

Or maybe you need to be reminded that happiness will not always predominate at the beginning, even when everything is normal.

"I Can't Cope with the Baby Right After the Birth"

The mother who gave birth to Adam could hardly bear to look at him when he was born. She was exhausted. She had experienced a difficult pregnancy, little sleep, 65 pounds extra weight, a couple of unruly boys at home. She was two weeks overdue, had a slow start, was induced with suppositories, and needed a hormone drip. I took part in inducing the labor and followed up with her the next day.

That mother was actually quite angry with her baby, she confided to me later. He hadn't even had the sense to arrive on time, and his hard head was "pretty painful" to deliver. She only glanced at him when told that he was a boy. If only he had been a little girl. Adam was boy number three—the same as the others, only even bigger. Massive. His skin was red and flaking because he had stayed in the amniotic fluid for so long after term. His square mouth simply bawled and demanded, just as the others had. His father had gone straight home to look after the big brothers.

The only thing she could think about was rest—now, when she was free from the others for a few days, in any case. She was free from bed-wetting and asthma and looked forward to sleep, relaxation. She could not cope with having her newborn baby on her belly, at the breast. She waved him away. He could wait. She figured she would give him the breast later on, but only while she was still in the hospital. These things had merely been a bother the other times. A bottle is easier because you can see what the baby is getting and don't have to worry about it.

CARE FOR THE MOTHER—SO SHE HAS STRENGTH FOR THE BABY

Adam's mother was sorely in need of care. Getting such care was perhaps easier in the old days, despite greater poverty. Until deliveries were hospitalized around the middle of the last century, friendly neighbors surrounded the woman giving birth, not only to help during the birth but also to help the new mother afterward. These other women looked after mother and child and cleaned the house, too. They made sure that the newcomer started to suckle, pacified a crying baby, and let the mother rest. They cooked meals, took care of the other children, and looked after the cow barn for the new mother. Relatives and neighbors came with gifts: a rich, home-cooked sour cream porridge (a traditional present when visiting a woman after childbirth in Norway) and other goodies. The mother usually lay on show—sometimes for weeks—with the baby next to her. Indeed, she got too much bed rest and for too long; quite a few of these new mothers ended up with blood clots. But at least they got their rest.

Then childbirth was institutionalized. Maternity clinics became common. Many older women today say that the only vacation they ever had was their stay in the maternity ward. Their voices get filled with longing when they talk about their lying in. Gradually, childbirth and confinement also came under the influence of German medicine. The baby was taken away from the mother for hygienic reasons, and newborn babies lay crowded in large nurseries, where they cried pitifully. The crying was so loud that people working there applied for a noise supplement to their pay. Scheduled feeding was introduced. The babies were weighed before and after a breastfeeding. They nursed from one breast every four hours. Breasts that could not adjust their production to being emptied every eight hours were declared unfit. This applied to most women who gave birth from after World War II until around 1975. Breastfeeding was more or less ruined for most of them.

But at least the new mothers had a week or two of rest and good nursing. Meals were served on the bedside table; while the women lay in bed, their genital areas were rinsed with soft soap and warm water several times a day, and visiting hours were strictly complied with. The mothers lay like queens and smiled politely among their flowers. But their breasts were overfull and felt like stones, and their ears pricked uneasily toward the howling in the nursery: "Is that my baby missing me? Who needs feeding? Who needs me?"

Today's mothers have their babies back. The maternity wards have become quiet, and only occasionally is the baby heard.

STARTING A GOOD CIRCLE

Adam's mother needed rest, good care, and respect for her feelings. She was worn out. The birth had been difficult, and the baby boy was not especially welcome. On top of that, Adam was not a baby with whom you immediately fell in love. He was bluish red with puffy eyes. The fact that Adam's mother was not immediately taken with her baby did not make her a bad mother. She was just a tired woman who was unenthusiastic about the situation at hand.

Because Adam's mother felt like this, though, she really needed everything that could link her closely to her little son. She needed the experience that the two of them belonged, for better or for worse. Whatever he was like, he was her baby. And even though she was worn out and angry and did not feel very much love immediately after the birth, she was still irreplaceable as the vitally important, unique mother to him.

The wise midwife who delivered Adam realized this. She let the mother recover after the birth and looked after her well. I was there and stayed for a while because there had been some complications along the way.

After a while, when the tears were stitched and the afterbirth had come out, the midwife said, "He's a bit cold. He needs body heat"— and without any further ado, she put Adam under his mother's covers. "But he might fall out of this narrow bed," the mother said in a tired voice, and she put an arm around him. "I've just got to go and get something," said the midwife, and she disappeared for a while. Later she came back and put Adam in the crib.

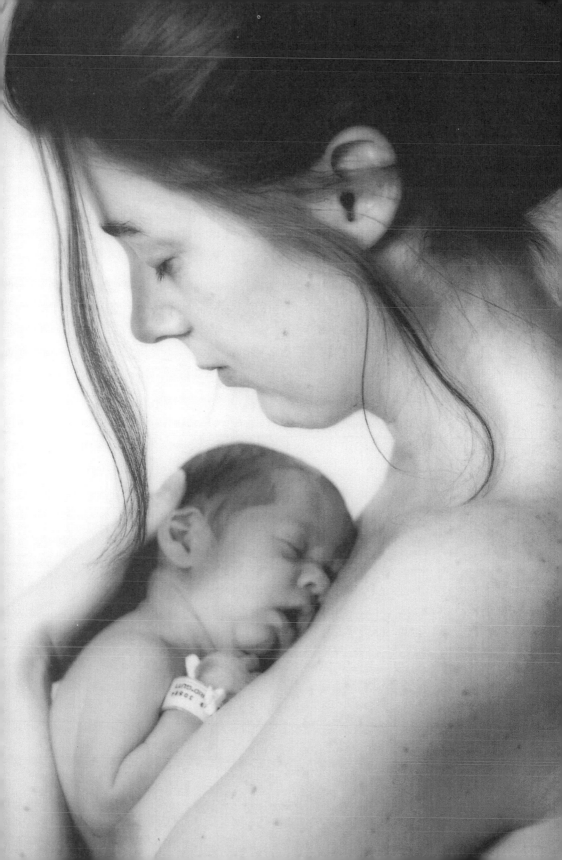

He started crying. After two slices of bread and some hot coffee, his mother said, "He sure is crying, isn't he?" The midwife answered, "Yes, I can't seem to quiet him. He calms down better with you." A tired, resigned smile, rather proud, appeared on the mother's face at this first little victory. "I guess he knows that I'm his mom," she said. Later she commented, "Look how he's struggling and sucking his hand." The midwife did not reply. "He must be hungry?"

Eventually Adam was put to the breast, gripped greedily, and sucked, looking like a cherub. "Now then," the midwife said, "perhaps that's enough. You'll want to rest, won't you?" There was a pause. "Oh, I don't know," the mother said. "He can stay a bit longer. None of the others tried so soon. Wow, how keen he is!" It was another little victory.

"Perhaps we've become more sensible on the maternity ward since the last time you were here," the midwife said. "The hospital used to enforce some really strange rules. Almost everyone breastfeeds here now, even women who thought it was a drag the first time around." She smiled. Adam fell asleep with the breast still in his mouth, and his mother, slightly lethargic from breastfeeding hormones, mumbled, "It's not that I don't want to. It's just that it mustn't be too stressful."

I sneaked out from my observation corner and thought to myself, "Perhaps the vicious circle has turned now. Perhaps this will be her favorite, the one who gives her confirmation that for him, she is Supermom. Maybe, just maybe, Mom's warm feelings and sense of achievement will benefit the other family members as well."

We who work with childbirth must try to feel our way carefully, giving care, support, and relief. At the same time, we must do everything we can to strengthen the mother-child relationship. It is particularly in those cases where conditions are a bit difficult that early bonding is important.

After six weeks, I saw Adam and his mother again. She had decided to be sterilized; she'd had enough babies. She was just as tired as before, with dark circles under her eyes. But she smiled quite tenderly at her baby, who lay in his stroller, when I asked whether everything was OK with him. "Yes," she replied. "You know, this little scoundrel is the first of my boys to get milk from just me. He won't have anything else. It's cheap, too. And it's quite restful during the day when I lie down and feed him. The others have to manage as best they can themselves, even if it sounds as though they're tearing the apartment down over my head."

Adam had become a wide-eyed, alert little baby. He looked as though he were immensely pleased with life and with his mother—for the time being, anyway.

"I Never Get Any Peace: The Baby Clings to Me and Eats Me Up"

"I just can't cope anymore. I'm falling apart!" exclaimed Charlotte, as she marched out. She smiles at the memory today, now with her second child, cuddling up with him, feeling that it's quite OK to be eaten up. She asked me to share with others the story of her first-born, however, because the desperation had come as a humbling shock at the time.

Charlotte was twenty-nine years old at the time. Everything was great: her education, her career, her marriage, a first baby planned. She had several years as an independent single woman behind her, was often out on the town, and spent a lot of time on personal style and care. An attractive woman she was.

That's why the change after the birth of her child had been too abrupt. All day long, a little creature had wanted to be close to her, crying, unhappy, demanding, wet. It was simply too much for her. Not just her breasts, but her whole personality was being sucked out of her, she said.

Fortunately, Charlotte's family had understood that she meant business. All had helped out so that she had several periods of a few hours to herself during the day. On nights when he was not working the next day, her husband slept with the baby in another room and brought the baby to Charlotte only when a feeding was needed. After a few weeks, Charlotte's desperation had gradually disappeared, but it returned every now and again during the first year. This is not uncommon.

Angry and Disappointed After Giving Birth?

"What do you really think about your delivery?" I often ask the new mothers when I do the rounds in the maternity ward. Many of them are very satisfied. Perhaps you are, too. The father of your baby was a warm rock to cling to along the way. The obstetrician and nurses were wise and close but had the good sense to stay away most of the time and respect the work the two of you were doing. You managed without much pain relief, and you think you got exactly the help you wanted. The birth, which recently stood out like a mountain and blocked the view beyond, has been conquered!

Frequently, however, I find that sympathetic questioning opens the floodgates. Pent-up frustration pours out. Feelings surface that did not seem quite permissible because there was so much to be grateful for. It can be important to know that you are not alone in having these feelings. Many women have highly negative feelings about their deliveries and subsequent care. Remember that your experiences and feelings are true for you. They are yours. You are allowed to feel like this. You have a right to bubble with happiness but also to be disappointed, angry, tired, and depressed.

Your feelings need to be acknowledged. You need to share them and be genuinely admired at what you have achieved—but you also need understanding about your sad, difficult feelings.

Perhaps you were disappointed? You were cheated of your major test of strength because it was decided that your baby should be delivered by cesarean section. The hospital took over; everything became technical and a bit frightening. Doctors brought your baby into the world, not you. Perhaps it took a long time before you got to see your baby properly after the operation. Maybe it hurt when that baby was finally put on your stomach following your recent operation.

Or perhaps you are furious? You feel cheated. Why didn't anyone actually prepare you for the fact that the birth would be the most painful experience you have ever had? Why did it take so terribly long? Why did no one help you? Why didn't they comfort you properly when you endured the contractions that drained you for hours? Why did the midwife disappear from the room just when you felt that you needed her most?

Why did your companion gradually become so unbelievably annoying and completely unable to understand what you were going through? How could he crunch on an apple or go out and read the newspaper while the contractions were tearing you apart? Or why did he hang over you the whole time, claiming that you were not breathing the way you had been taught in Lamaze class, almost massaging a hole in your back, splashing about with a wet cloth when you wanted only to drift off and lie there for a bit between contractions?

Why didn't anyone understand that you were actually quite embarrassed and thought that it was dreadful to have your private parts exposed unnecessarily? A little consideration would have gone a long way. Had they no idea that you felt like a beached whale lying huge and heavy and naked and having to roll around on that hard delivery bed—with needles in your arm, a plastic tube in your back, a catheter in your bladder, an electrode on the baby's head inside your vagina, and a belt to record the contractions around your stomach?

Why did no one look after your dignity? And your sweetheart: will he ever be able to look at you romantically again after all this, after all the urine and excrement and blood and amniotic fluid, and the cutting and sewing of your most private parts, which only you and he had known before?

Or perhaps you are still worn out by the worry itself, the concern about everything that was going to happen to you. Would you manage to keep your composure? Would you behave like a real woman, like an Earth Mother? How on Earth was it possible that a big baby's head—4 inches from ear to ear, the doctor had said—could get through your tight opening, which was suddenly supposed to function as the gateway to life? What about the worry that something would be wrong with the baby? Why was the midwife so hectic, and why did she call the doctor? They kept studying the long strips of paper and muttering with their backs to you. Suddenly you were told to breathe oxygen. Why did they press your abdomen and fuss and call out?

Why did the doctor's face turn red from exhaustion when he was trying to get the baby out, nearly dragging you off the bed in the process? And that limp, bluish thing that you delivered—didn't it look kind of dead? When suddenly the screaming started, the baby still didn't look quite right. Maybe you had done a poor job of pushing and you had injured the baby? Even though it all turned out perfectly well, you are still worried, and the joy you expected to feel just is not there.

Perhaps you had decided beforehand not to have any pain-relief medication. You felt inside that you would be up to the great "birthing test," and now you are wondering whether you failed. The birth was to be like a marathon race, tough, painful at times, but victory would come at the end. Instead, you hung onto the mask with laughing gas all the time, or you were injected full of pethidine or Demorol. The contractions were so dreadfully painful along the way, and then when the midwife came with the syringe, you said yes with immense gratitude.

Everyone around you seemed to believe that you fared a little better than you actually did. Personally, you feel that the only difference was that you became incredibly sick and sleepy, while the contractions were just as painful. Now they came rolling down on you like a nightmare, without you being properly awake and able to tackle them at all.

You are quite right. Although pethidine and Demerol, which resembles morphine, do make you lethargic, they do not actually help relieve the pains of childbirth. Some women need the relaxing effect, but they need to be told that the injection is for this purpose, not to take away the pain. It is also good to know the side effects of pethidine so that you will understand their cause if they occur. Many women feel nauseated, unwell, or dizzy when given the medication. In addition, pethidine has a dulling effect on the baby. Only about half of all new-born babies affected by pethidine spontaneously take the initiative to search for the breast, thus getting breastfeeding off to a good start. The other half spend days mustering enough energy to suck, and they can be sleepy and listless. Pethidine can in fact remain in the baby for weeks after the birth. This condition will pass, but the breastfeeding will probably require extra effort for a time.

Or perhaps you are cross with yourself because you ended up with an epidural, something you had never imagined? You believed deep inside yourself that only sissies needed the epidural. So now you are a sissy, too? Far from it!

Deliveries vary enormously. Especially if labor has lasted for many hours, most women need pain relief beyond what is available through traditional means, such as warm baths, backrubs, heat, and pethidine. In the best cases, modern epidurals are so finely adjusted that you can move your legs, feel the contractions, and push the baby out yourself. But this is not always true. Sometimes you are almost paralyzed for a few hours, unable even to urinate unaided, and you need help getting the baby out.

Remember that a difficult birth this time does not mean that the next time will be equally hard as well. On the contrary, most women find that the first birth is the most difficult, not least because it often takes so long.

It may help to talk through the events of the birth with the midwife or the doctor who was there. You will not always get the support you need, however. The midwife you were so happy about may be off duty after a night shift. The doctor may have come for a quick visit but then been called away posthaste. The nurse who was so nice after the birth may be nowhere to be seen.

Don't be afraid to ask for the people you want to see again. Someone should listen to your feelings. As a rule, the staff want to visit the mothers whose births they attended, but this may get overlooked during a busy workday. Sometimes only a little reminder is needed; at other times, a shift change or time off prevent the follow-up visit.

The goal is for the person who helped your baby into the world to sit down and talk through the birth with you. If this is not possible, ask another staff member to find the notes describing the birth and to come and sit with you while you talk and ask questions. If even this proves impossible, ask to come back again after a while—perhaps for a six-week checkup—and talk about what you want to know about your delivery then. Painful birth experiences sometimes become so effectively buried after a while that you do not remember them until the next time you are pregnant. You can also talk about your painful birth experiences then. It's never too late.

Through your experiences, we medical staff can also become wiser and more competent. Share them with us even if we seem busy at the time.

Baby Blues

Even when you are completely satisfied with the birth and your baby, your emotions can give you an unpleasant surprise after a few days. Elisabeth had heard about the down days, or "baby blues." She didn't think that they would affect her. She felt energetic and happy after the birth: excited. Her tummy was flat again, the longed-for princess took well to her breast, and the flowers came flooding in. She was so pleased when I talked with her the day after the birth, happy over a healthy baby and a nice husband who looked forward to having them home. Everyone was being so nice; everything was going so well.

Then, two days later, I was called to see her. The nurses were at a loss. Elisabeth just cried. She lay with the covers over her head and could not explain what was wrong. The problem was actually that nothing was wrong. Or everything. Life was just bearing down on her. Eventually, she managed to put some of it into words. How would she cope with the responsibility for her baby? The busy nurse who had been a bit brusque in the morning had become a monster. Someone had hinted that the baby was a bit yellow. Even if they said "quite normal," could she rely on this? And was Dan really happy about her the way she looked now, fat and ugly and with tangled hair, leaking breasts, and bleeding genitals? Perhaps he was out looking for another woman? And why had she been so horrid to her mother while in her teens? Now she knew what it was to bring a baby into the world. Just think if her own child turned out to be so ungrateful!

What in the world had happened to Elisabeth? The baby blues had hit her. Many women experience something like this, and I think that the explanation includes several factors.

First, the pregnancy hormones are in free fall. During pregnancy, the placenta produced huge quantities of the female sex hormones estrogen and progesterone. These are the same hormones that fluctuate during the menstrual cycle. Suddenly the whole of the large placenta is gone, and with it, the hormones. The change can feel like a very sudden case of menopause. Immediately after the birth, most women are excited and in a good mood if they have not had too difficult a time. They want to cuddle their baby, talk with their husband, remember the birth, listen to praise about their efforts, and thank those who helped. This may be connected to the fact that during birth a woman produces her own painkilling pleasure hormones, endorphins. These hormones stay in her system for a while and can certainly contribute to her heightened mood. In addition, the adrenaline she has produced causes excitement.

This is appropriate, to start with at any rate. Something similar occurs in other mammals. The female does not give birth and then lie down to sleep straight away. She actively clears up traces of blood and the afterbirth and makes sure that the young is breathing, moves about, and gets to the nipples. If necessary, she takes herself and her offspring to safety before she rests.

I once sat in the pen of a nanny goat who had just given birth to a kid that had something wrong with it. The goat was kind, motherly, and experienced. When she had licked and fiddled about with the kid for a while and it gave no signs of getting up, she began to stimulate it. She nudged it and moved it around but got no reaction. She scraped with increasing intensity at the young one with her cloven hooves. The kid tried to get up. It couldn't. The goat nudged it, and it looked as though she offered the udder, tempted it. Still there was no effect. Finally the nanny goat became quite brutal, scraping and kicking the helpless kid again and again until the farmer came and tried to help. The kid died during the night. After the birth, the nanny goat had known instinctively that something had to be done. If the young one did not do what it was supposed to do, it was sentenced to doom.

Sometimes I wonder whether some of the same instincts play havoc in women who have just given birth. Some are almost hyperactive immediately after the delivery. But then comes the downturn. Slowly the new mother begins to realize what the baby will demand, this little being with a right to a full twenty-four-hour service. There will be sleepless nights, responsibility. You become extra vulnerable when you have not had much sleep—but disturbed nights are a part of having a new baby.

The first few days are often tiring. Two unknown people have to become familiar with each other's behavior. Maybe the mother thinks her baby does not like her. She feels that the baby is rejecting her, crying inconsolably or having problems taking the breast at the beginning. Or maybe the mother has not fallen in love with her baby yet and fears that she will not be a good mother. She may even be a bit disappointed about the baby's appearance or behavior.

We don't usually find one obvious explanation for these baby blues. They generally appear three to ten days after the birth. One should not scorn or ignore them. What can be done is for the mother to be pampered. The staff made sure that Elisabeth got plenty of rest, good food, and lots to drink. She took a long afternoon nap every day. She received extra attention for her relatively minor problems with regard to breastfeeding, constipation, and pain. She was comforted and told that the feelings would soon pass—and they usually do. Two days later, Elisabeth beamed again and felt full of confidence that everything would work out.

Postpartum Depression and Psychosis

Women who have given birth may also experience more serious depression. This seems to be a good deal more common than previously believed. Life becomes gray. The mother feels down and sad, always tired, often sleepless, constantly despairing, and unhappy about the baby. She may benefit from counseling and, in some cases, medication against depression. Dealing with depression can take a long time and also makes demands on those close to her. Both she and the baby will benefit from the active participation of other people, however.

Occasionally, a woman develops a postpartum psychosis with delusions. She may be convinced that someone—or she herself—wants to kill the baby, for example. She may be confused and full of anxiety, feeling that someone wants to hurt her. She may see and hear things that do not exist. She is unable to take responsibility for herself and the baby, struggles to sleep, and may express a wish to take her own life. Postpartum psychosis is a serious mental illness. The few women who develop postpartum psychosis have, as a rule, been especially psychologically vulnerable beforehand. In addition, they have often been exposed to extra strain during pregnancy and childbirth. They are commonly relatively alone in the world, without a good support network. The most serious cases require admission to a psychiatric hospital. But most women do recover.

Such a psychosis or long-term depression must not be confused with normal baby blues. We must not make illnesses out of common reactions to life crises, which first and foremost require someone to talk with, to care, and to provide.

Happiness is commonly a long time in coming for new mothers, especially when:

- You are extremely tired.

- The birth was unusually difficult.

- The hormone changes are at their worst, after a few days.

- The big responsibility suddenly becomes real to you.

- The baby has to stay in a pediatric ward.

- The baby cries inconsolably most of the time.

- You have difficulty getting breastfeeding started.

- You are worried about the baby.

- You feel exhausted with another being next to you most of the time.

- You have had previous problems with depression or anxiety.

CHAPTER 6

• • •

After Cesarean, Forceps, or Vacuum Delivery

Delivery by cesarean section is one common reason for a baby's less-than-ideal start to life. Sonia and Kim gave birth with a planned cesarean section on the same day at the same hospital. Each woman was given an epidural spinal anesthetic, both had their partner with them, and both had lovely healthy sons. But the two women had very different experiences.

SONIA'S DISAPPOINTMENT

After his birth, Sonia's little boy was immediately carried out of the operating room. Later, the midwife returned and showed him to his parents. Mostly only his father could see him then; the angle wasn't quite right for Sonia. She actually saw only a bit of hair and the tip of a nose inside a blanket. The midwife and the baby then disappeared, with the father behind them. They were going to weigh, measure, and bathe the baby.

Sonia remained lying on the operating table surrounded by people she did not know. It seemed an eternity before the rest of the operation was completed. She had not been prepared for the fact that removing the placenta, stopping the bleeding, and sewing up the layers would take longer than it took to get the baby out. She had a little pain, or maybe it was mostly tension? It helped a bit, at any rate, when her anesthesiologist chatted with her during the process.

Wide awake, full of expectation, and free of pain, Sonia was moved to a postoperative ward. There she felt a pang of disappointment when she learned that she would not be able to see her baby during the two hours she needed to stay there, because she shared the room with other people who had recently undergone operations, including one who had just been operated on for blocked fallopian tubes causing infertility.

In the meantime, the baby screamed inconsolably on a completely different floor. The new father's slightly clumsy attempt to comfort him did not help much. Because the father was also quite busy calling relatives and friends, the staff looked in on the little boy at regular intervals, but they had a lot of other things to do as well. By the time Sonia finally got her baby for herself, he was several hours old. He slept from exhaustion and hardly woke again that day; the last thing he wanted to do was to suck at her breast.

KIM'S JOY

Kim, who was operated on that same afternoon in that same hospital, had initially been disappointed when she had learned that her pelvis was too narrow for a vaginal delivery of her baby. She had read about birth and the period just afterward, had seen a video, and gone to pre-natal class. She told me the day before the birth that she was looking forward with great joy to the first encounter with her baby. It had been decided that I would perform the cesarean section. It is always a good idea to talk things through in advance, and because Kim was so disappointed about not being able to deliver vaginally, we decided to make the first meeting with the baby as positive as possible. We would try to help fulfill Kim's dreams. In this case, good cooperation was required from the midwife present, the operating nurses, and, not least, the anesthetist and anesthetic nurse. Quite a few people cooperate during a cesarean section.

Kim had her epidural. Everything worked out perfectly. She heard her little boy's cry as soon as I lifted him carefully from her womb. After his umbilical cord had been cut, I held him up for a moment above the screen that separated the operating area from Kim's head, where the father sat and the anesthesia staff worked. Sure enough, the little boy peed straight into his mother's face, while both parents marveled, smiling over their wet, slightly purple, wriggling son. He was then handed over to the midwife, who carried him into the side room, dried him well, and checked that everything was OK and that he was breathing normally.

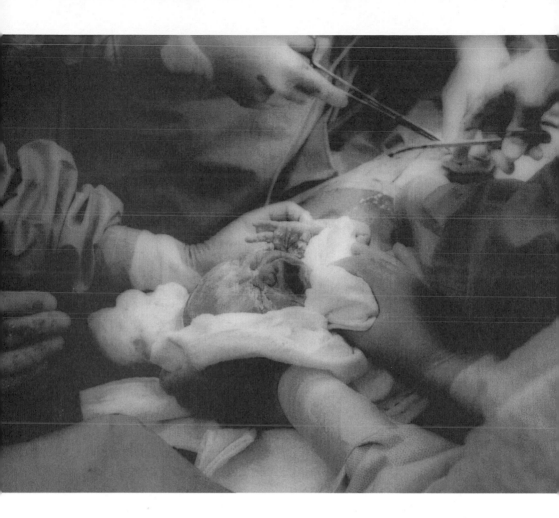

Wrapped in warm blankets, the baby was returned to the operating room. His father held him first for a moment, up to his mother's face. She sniffed and kissed him, cried and laughed. Then her shirt was unbuttoned, and the little boy's blanket was opened before he was placed skin-to-skin across Kim's chest. Covered with blankets, he soon relaxed on his mother's warm chest to the sounds from her heart. Then began what Kim afterward called the golden rendezvous with her baby. The whole time, she had a caressing hand under the baby blanket.

The little fellow called out, and his mother answered him; his father smiled with moist eyes. Amazingly, by the time we had finished the operation, the baby had found his own way to the nipple and had begun to suck eagerly. The midwife watched from afar; the anesthesia staff quietly checked their tasks. The baby was left with his mother until the last stitch had been inserted with the almost-invisible thread that closes the skin and gradually disappears by itself.

After a short separation while Kim was moved to the recovery room, she was again given her baby, and they continued where they had left off. The father sat with them, responsible for watching the baby and returning him to the maternity ward if he cried too much so that he would not disturb the other patients who had been recently operated on. But hardly a sound came from the newborn boy.

Kim was moved to the maternity ward after a few hours. The little family had been together nearly the whole time, and everyone was immensely pleased. The baby boy had been allowed to follow his instincts, been allowed to suck for as long as he wanted. He had received some valuable, protective drops of mother's milk before he fell into the deep, long sleep that characterizes many newborn babies after their first wide-awake hours.

The childless woman who had recently been operated on still lay behind the screens in the same monitoring room. She could make out what was going on, listening to small sounds and a little crying. I had talked with her before the baby was brought in, and she felt it was OK with her.

"Anyway," she said afterward, "babies are everywhere. In some ways, this was encouraging. Perhaps it will be my turn next time."

Tell Them What You Want

Following a cesarean section at an obstetric department designated as "Baby-Friendly" as part of the WHO/UNICEF Initiative for successful breastfeeding, the mother has a right to be given her baby within half an hour after she can relate to it. This means as soon as is feasible after an epidural anesthesia, preferably on the operating table, as happened with Kim.

Getting the mother and baby together so quickly after a cesarean is not always possible, however. Several prerequisites must be fulfilled: the baby must be in good shape, the mother must not be in pain or have other problems, the surgeon must have been asked beforehand. A cesarean section is a major operation. The doctors who operate can encounter complications that require total concentration, and a baby placed on the mother's breast leaves less room for us to work on our side of the screen. The midwife who receives the newborn from the doctor must also be willing to stay in the operating room and look after the baby. This can sometimes interfere with other work needed in a busy maternity ward, but as a rule, the midwife is more than willing. A birth, whether natural or by cesarean section, does not normally end until the baby is sucking at the breast. Getting to this point is the midwife's responsibility, if circumstances allow.

Achieving such a meeting between mother and baby during or immediately after the operation, when possible, has many advantages. Allowing mother and baby to get to know each other, which seems to be ideal immediately after the birth, is only one of the benefits. In addition, the baby is able to practice sucking while interest and sucking strength are at a peak. The breasts are stimulated at the time when they are most receptive and receive powerful signals to start producing milk.

Stimulation of the breasts leads to a surge of oxytocin to the womb, which helps the womb to contract properly. Recently I stood with a limp, bleeding uterus between my hands during a cesarean section. We had given an artificial hormone, as we always do in such situations, but the womb had not reacted as desired. Suddenly, however, it became firm and hard, and the bleeding stopped. Astonished, I asked the anesthesiologist whether he had administered extra medication without my request. He had not. Instead, the midwife had placed the baby on the breast of the mother, and suddenly the baby had found her own way and started to suck, bringing about good hormonal response. The timing may have been coincidental, but the effect was impressive. It makes one wonder whether the oxytocin produced by the mother herself at times works better than the synthetic one.

Many women who are awake during a cesarean section feel discomfort from the operation. Anxiety or boredom always reinforces this. The anesthesiological staff know this and are skilled at talking with the patient to distract her. Time and time again, I have found that the best diversion is to give the baby to the mother until the operation is over. It is sometimes funny to realize that while we are standing over the open belly, with bloody organs between our hands, the mother is lying happily chatting with her baby behind the screen.

When Dad Becomes the Welcoming Committee

This is also a good arrangement for the father, because he can be with both mother and baby at once. Many fathers are doubtful about where they belong if the midwife leaves with the baby. They enjoy being with the baby, watching the weighing and bathing, following everything that happens. At the same time, the father is really there for his partner's sake. He might feel uncomfortable leaving her while she is anxious in these slightly frightening and unknown surroundings.

Some women are fully anesthetized during a cesarean section— because they have chosen this themselves, because time does not allow for an epidural, or for other good reasons. In this situation, the father is not present during the operation. It takes a while before the woman comes around and is aware enough to rejoice over the baby. Some are very drowsy for hours, especially if they have a lot of pain when they wake up and need strong painkillers. Regardless of this, a mother has a right to have her baby with her as soon as she can relate to that baby, whether after one hour or four. If the mother longs for the baby while anesthesia still affects her, someone needs to sit with them both and look after them. Hospital staff are often too busy to help with this. And what is more natural than having the new father there? Most fathers do a brilliant job of looking after their baby and seeking help if needed.

Sometimes father and baby wait for a long time together before the mother comes around properly. Then I usually go to them when the operation is finished. We help the father into a rocking chair, unbutton his shirt, and unwrap the baby a bit before placing the infant on the father's chest. A father's body heat and heartbeat comfort many babies, although it is heartrending to see the baby struggle to find the promised feeding station, which the father doesn't have. Many fathers become quite moved in such a situation. They blush, look a bit warm and overwhelmed, and smile confusedly. Some babies actually grab hold of the hair on their father's chest, their grip reflex triggered when the hair touches the palms of their hands. This reflex, found only in quite young babies, is like that of newborn apes holding onto their mother's fur.

A useful trick if the mother cannot put the baby to her breast in the first few hours after birth is to stimulate her breasts in other ways, outside of the hospital gown. One can stroke, massage, roll, or rub the nipple. Anything that makes the nipple become firm and hard will help. If the mother cannot manage to do this herself, the father is again a natural and usually very willing partner. Such stimulation makes the breasts react extra well to the fact that a baby has been born and will soon need feeding; it is now only a matter of starting to produce milk. At the same time, oxytocin secreted during nipple stimulation makes the womb contract, which is particularly useful in the hours after the operation.

Some women who have had an epidural during a cesarean section continue to get needed pain relief via an epidural pump in the days after the operation. This helps control severe pain. Women without an epidural pump—especially women who are fully anesthetized during the operation—need other painkillers. Although all medicines will pass into the milk and can affect the baby slightly, such small quantities of milk are produced at this time that no danger is involved. By the time the quantity of milk increases, after a few days, the need for painkillers is normally much less. As a rule, breastfeeding goes very well by then, but a mother with a cesarean section may need a lot of extra help taking care of the baby and herself and later her home.

Most women are not very interested in food and drink after the operation. They need peace and quiet to recover. But mother and baby also need each other. The baby's crib should be positioned so that the mother can see her baby's face. Resourceful staff should be able to help find a breastfeeding position that does not make the operation wound hurt. It is often uncomfortable for a woman who has been recently operated on to turn from side to side to allow the baby to suck from both of her breasts. It can be a good idea to lie on the most comfortable side, place the baby on a cushion, and feed from the top breast first. Then pull the cushion away from beneath the baby so that the baby can suck on the bottom breast. This requires minimal effort and causes minimal discomfort for the mother.

Healthy women gradually recover after a cesarean section, and most feel able to go home after five to seven days. Some are particularly weary, for example, after losing an unusually large amount of blood or after complications such as cystitis or a wound infection with a fever. If there is capacity in the ward, it is wise for these women to stay as long as possible. Even if the mother is longing to go home, it is often difficult to get expert help there. An extra day or two in the hospital can make the difference as to whether she feels able to go up and down stairs and look after the baby herself. Breastfeeding also improves with each day.

Back home, it is sensible to stay in bed for a while with the baby at your side. The mother should rest and breastfeed and let others take care of everything else. A cesarean section has a much bigger impact on the body than does a normal delivery. No one expects a man who has had a major abdominal operation to run around and work in the first few weeks afterward.

After Forceps or Vacuum Delivery

Sometimes a delivery takes longer than is desirable because of the baby's position. Or the baby shows signs of becoming so exhausted at the end of the delivery that help is needed to complete the birth before the mother manages to push out the baby herself. In these cases, the baby is often delivered using forceps or a suction cup with a vacuum.

The vaginal opening is more likely to be cut in these cases than when the delivery is spontaneous, and extra tears are common. These must be sewn up carefully. Afterward, both mother and baby are usually particularly exhausted. The experience often has been long and tiring, and the end may have been a bit dramatic. Perhaps a pediatrician needs to check the baby. These things can mean postponement of the satisfying start with the baby on the mother's belly. As soon as mother and baby are able, this relationship should be initiated exactly as after any other birth.

When the baby is delivered by cesarean section, you can ask:

- For the baby to be put on your chest during the operation if you are awake.

- For the baby to be positioned so that you can look into the eyes.

- For the baby to be brought to you in the recovery room when you want.

- For the baby to be able to lie skin-to-skin with you as soon as is feasible.

- For the baby to stay with you for as long as you want.

- For the dad or another person to sit by your bed and take responsibility for the baby.

- For assistance with helping the baby to latch onto your breast as soon as the baby is ready to do so.

- For frequent help with breastfeeding from the first day onward if you want it.

- For help with alternative breastfeeding positions that do not make the operation wound hurt.

- For lots of support and relief at the time surrounding the birth; your job is to recover and breastfeed your baby.

CHAPTER 7

· · ·

When Mother and Baby Are Separated

Tiny Peter appeared far too early—more than ten weeks before he was due. There was no stopping his early arrival. An unfinished creature of just over 2 pounds, he needed help breathing and was immediately dealt with by a pediatrician. A semi-rigid tube was inserted into his airway and connected to a respirator. He had to be placed in an incubator and was immediately transferred to the special care unit for newborn babies.

In the delivery room, Peter's mother was left with empty arms. There was no eager little mouth, no warm, nuzzling bundle as a reward for the effort. She felt only worry: would he be all right? He was so small! Several hours later, she and her husband were sitting next to the incubator, but that was not exactly reassuring. She said afterward that Peter reminded her of a skinned rabbit, because of the thin, transparent skin through which his blood shone red. Or he seemed like a little hedgehog with tubes and wires sticking out everywhere. It was not easy to decide whether he was sweet or not. The breathing tube was stuck with adhesive tape to his chin so that his little face looked completely distorted. There were no open blue eyes to gaze into; the mother could not possibly smell or pat the baby or offer the breast or other skin contact.

Peter's parents had heard how important close contact and breastfeeding were from the beginning. Now, though, their baby was enclosed in a plastic box, less accessible than he had been in the womb. At least then, they could feel him kicking and know that he was OK. A sense of sadness set in.

In contrast to Peter, Katherine was born on her due date at a local hospital. She weighed almost 9 pounds and was big and strong. After a few hours, though, she was rushed to the pediatric unit at the University hospital because she had turned blue and was experiencing increasing trouble breathing. A heart defect that had to be operated on was diagnosed. Katherine's young mother was transferred to our postnatal unit at the same time. Here there were only unknown staff; no family or friends were close by.

Katherine's mother made her way to the ward for pediatric surgery and sat there for much of the day, full of dark thoughts. Later, she talked about worrying that she had done something wrong during the pregnancy to cause Katherine to be born with a defect—and a heart defect at that. She wondered if this could have happened because she had not felt warmhearted toward the baby, had not really wanted Katherine. She felt too young and had an unstable relationship with the baby's father. She had hoped that a sweet little baby would bring them closer together. Instead, even this had gone wrong.

Now she sat alone, and I thought that she in particular could have used the best start possible to bond emphatically with her baby, to experience herself as a natural, successful mother from the first moment.

Laura also arrived on time, but toward the end of the delivery, her heart beat very slowly. Because she lacked oxygen, she had her first bowel movement into the amniotic fluid, and she was so unlucky as to get some of it into her lungs. She was suctioned as well as possible when she was born, but she struggled to breathe and was transferred to the pediatric unit for observation. Her parents worried.

Eric's mother, in contrast, was so ill herself that she hardly registered what was going on during the birth of her baby. She had preeclamptic toxemia, with a blood pressure that rose and rose. This affected the placenta, causing Eric to grow slowly. Finally, her condition became so threatening that the baby was delivered prematurely by cesarean section. Eric was a small, undernourished, grayish creature, and his mother was doing so poorly that she had to be specially monitored for many days. Eric's father commuted anxiously between the two wards.

These are just some of the many sad cases in the maternity ward. Sometimes you feel completely torn between the greatest happiness in one room and the deepest sorrow in the next. If time allows in such situations, I pause, draw a deep breath, and switch gears, so to speak.

Fortunately, most babies are born healthy and at full term. That makes it all the harder for the ones who are not so lucky. Everything eventually went well in the four cases just mentioned—but rivers of tears and sweat flowed in the meantime.

How to Overcome a Difficult Start

Dear Mom and Dad who have had such hurtful experiences after having a baby: Of course you feel unhappy and despairing. Life is unfair. In addition to experiencing a traumatic medical problem with your baby, you missed out on an exciting start with a healthy, full-term, almost self-sufficient baby who set in motion many kinds of positive processes. I hope that someone will look after you lovingly and tell you that you can do a lot for your baby even when temporarily separated.

Remember that everything is not lost, even if you don't have an ideal start. Humans with their big brains are designed to bond with each other in many ways. Parents of adopted children know a lot about this. The capacity for repair is great, and there will be good opportunities to make up for what is missed.

Find out what is best for your baby, even if your heart breaks a little when what you find is far from what you expected. Simply use your head and intuition and give whatever contact you can, depending on the baby's condition.

Visit the baby as soon as possible, and stay in the ward as much as you can. You have a right to be in the pediatric ward for most of the day. Even if you are ill or have been recently operated on, you can be wheeled in to visit your baby.

You may feel inadequate with your baby surrounded by experts specially trained in taking care of newborn babies with problems. This expertise is needed, but your baby also needs stable, loving parents nearby, and the staff can never replace you. Think about this if you feel bored and tired, being there a lot without anything special to do.

Perhaps your baby cannot bear being touched for a while. A baby who should still be lying protected in the mother's womb needs a lot of peace. Sit down, talk softly, or sing a little song. The baby will recognize mother's and perhaps father's voice and will need to become even more familiar with these voices. They represent the stability that will follow through thick and thin for many years.

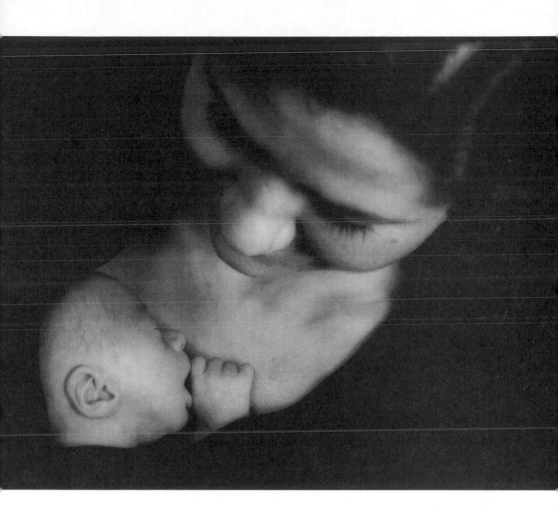

You can usually pat your baby a little quite early on, or just sit with one hand nearby, quite peacefully. You have the time and patience and will quickly become experts on what is good for your own baby. The staff will change shifts and have many babies to look after. Ask when you are in doubt, but use your intuition. Perhaps you will find that stroking a little hand with a loving finger will quiet your baby, or that a little cautious patting on the bottom will make your baby sleep.

Some nurses make a small, soft nest around the baby in the incubator and are clever at shielding the infant from unnecessary noise and light. Others are perhaps not so concerned about this. Ask for your baby to be protected like this all the time if you notice that it seems to have a soothing effect. You see your baby every day. Perhaps you can help to build the nest yourself.

Let your baby smell your clean hands. As the mother, rub your fingers on the tip of your breast first; the glands there secrete a scent that are attractive to your baby. Or express a little milk on your finger; the baby can smell this even if not ready to eat anything yet.

MOTHER'S MILK WITHOUT BREASTFEEDING

The staff will want to give a sick or premature baby a little breast milk within hours of birth, a few milliliters at a time, more as medicine than as food. This milk protects the baby against a number of diseases and complications and at the same time sets in motion a maturing process for the bowel.

If the baby cannot yet swallow, the breast milk is given through a probe—a thin, soft plastic tube that goes directly down into the stomach. A little breast milk and stimulation are also good for the mouth. In many hospitals, the mother and father use a cotton swab, dip it in breast milk, and brush it inside the baby's mouth and on the lips. It is touching to see how eager the baby can become.

To do this, you need some milk to give to the baby, preferably as soon as possible. Producing this milk is not easy when you are perhaps upset and anxious and when you have been deprived of the strong signals from the baby's early sucking.

Relax! It will be OK! The strongest signal for milk production is simply that the afterbirth has come away. During pregnancy, the placental hormones prevent much milk from being produced. Anyone who has had a baby will get milk in her breasts.

But the earlier and the clearer the signals received by the breast, the better they respond. If you have enough strength to think about this immediately after the birth, perhaps because you expected what happened, it may be wise for you to use your hands to stimulate your breasts. In this way, you "dupe" your breasts into sending signals about hormone production, and milk production is speeded up. You can read about this in chapter 6.

If the baby is not put to the breast for a day or two, you must start pumping or hand-expressing your milk. You will receive advice about this in both the maternity ward and the pediatric ward. Research has shown that you should pump your breasts for a total of two or more hours per day, divided into five or six times, for stable and adequate milk production. After you have learned how to pump, ask whether someone can teach you to do double pumping, which increases the breastfeeding hormones and the milk quantity and allows you to cut down on your pumping time.

Many women become fed up with pumping. A common complaint goes something like this: "I feel like a cow at a milking machine. When the others have their babies at the breast, I'm blubbering in the pump room." At the same time, most women are highly motivated to do this because they know that sick, disabled, or premature babies especially need breast milk.

Many mothers find hand-expression of milk faster and more straightforward than pumping. There are a few tricks to this, but most women find it works well after a couple of times. Study hand-expression in a video such as *Breast Is Best,* which also shows a small, premature baby suckling for the first time. The video is available in many hospitals and at health centers. (See Resources, page 253.)

Eventually, you will have your baby lying on your chest, out of the incubator. In the special care unit, you often have to be satisfied initially with the little one lying peacefully there, listening, smelling, and enjoying the time out. Ask to be allowed to hold your baby as much as possible; the contact is usually good for all parties.

Should complications or a long-term separation prohibit breast-feeding, the baby will, in most hospitals, be given breast milk from a milk bank, possibly together with additional nutrients. In a breast milk bank, surplus milk from healthy, non-smoking, non-medicated women is frozen after extensive testing, and later used for premature babies and other high-risk infants in pediatric wards.

Even if you can't breastfeed, you can still give plenty of contact and care. One particularly satisfying method for parents to interact with sick babies originated with "kangaroo babies" in South America. In poor countries there, where incubators and special care are not readily affordable, small premature babies are put between their mother's breasts, under her clothes. The baby lives there all the time. The baby's bottom is wiped when appropriate, and a breast is stuck into the mouth whenever the baby whimpers or is willing to take it. There is no stress or tiring care, and the baby remains in the even body temperature of the mother. This works incredibly well.

This method should be used far more in rich countries as well, together with and in addition to our advanced postnatal medicine. If you have a premature baby who does not need a respirator and is old enough to coordinate sucking, swallowing, and breathing, you could ask to try this kangaroo method. Even when the baby is still on a respirator and too young to breastfeed, you can usually do it for parts of the day. Feeding directly from the breast is usually possible at around thirty-two to thirty-three weeks, about seven to eight weeks before the baby should have been born.

SUCKING FROM THE BREAST IS EVENTUALLY ALLOWED

Sooner or later, the baby is ready for the breast. An exciting moment ensues. Breastfeeding can best happen quite undramatically, with the baby smelling, tasting, and sucking and not being expected to drink much milk. Often, in fact, the baby is put to the breast while still being fed through a tube. In this way, the infant learns to associate the breast with a feeling of fullness and well-being. This is a good starting point from which the growing baby may gradually take more and more from the breast until that wonderful day when nothing else is needed.

Here is some other good advice for caring for weak babies: They must not be stressed, but should instead be stimulated. A weak baby often sucks best with its body tucked under the mother's arm; the baby's head must often be specially supported in her hand. Ask for help, and count on needing a lot of time to practice. Check that your baby is eventually put to the breast before being given pumped milk or formula, and be prepared for the fact that your baby's weight may remain static for a few days after you finally dare to take the step to full breastfeeding.

The first really good meeting is sometimes simply when the baby is discharged to the maternity ward after short-term observation in the pediatric ward, perhaps after a few days. Make sure that you have peace and quiet. Take the baby under the covers with you. Unbutton your shirt, undress at least the baby's upper body, and place the baby on your naked skin.

Wait patiently. After a while, the baby, often slowly, will begin to recover some of what was missed immediately after birth. Your little one will snuffle, stretch, and search. The baby should be neither full nor desperately hungry, but awake and interested. Massage the baby's back, smell and kiss the little head, have a cuddle. Given time, you and your baby will eventually find that both of you recover some of what you lost. Your wounds at being separated will gradually heal. Remember that this may take time for you as well. You will not necessarily feel pleasure or be overwhelmed with happiness right away by doing this—but try all the same.

Perhaps the story of little Boris will inspire you.

THE STORY OF LITTLE BORIS

The setting was the pediatric ward in Saint Petersburg, Russia, in the 1990s. Newborn babies there were still swaddled and kept in a building separate from their mothers. A small train of babies lying shoulder-to-shoulder, on shelves on top of each other, came at specific, infrequent times for feeding. Routines there were much the same as they had been in Norway in the 1960s. Scandinavian breastfeeding experts were visiting, running workshops, teaching how a change of routines could better encourage breastfeeding without costing a penny. This was important in a poor country where mothers gave their babies expensive formula because they believed the Russian women had lost the ability to breastfeed. This was just what women all over the Western world were led to believe thirty to fifty years ago—and what many still believe in places.

The staff was defensive and slightly aggressive. "Perhaps you can do something with Boris? He is several days old. He cries most of the time, won't suck at the breast, rejects the bottle, and is losing weight."

Boris looked like a tiny mummy, but with a square mouth that cried and cried, thin and dejected, fretting. "What about undressing him and putting him skin-to-skin with his mother?" suggested Anna-Berit Arvidson, a Swedish midwife. Slightly irritated, suspicious, scornful glances came from the Russian doctors and midwives.

Boris was unwound from his swaddling strips. His small arms came into view, free for his mother to see the first time since birth. His mother's shirt was unbuttoned, without anyone asking her for permission or explaining what was going on. Stark naked, frightened, with flailing arms and legs, Boris was placed on his mother's body.

Nothing happened. The crowd around the bed was restless. "And how long will this take?" asked the Russians, via the interpreter.

"It's difficult to say. Perhaps an hour, perhaps several days."

It took four minutes! Suddenly it was evident that little Boris sensed and sniffed. His arms and legs worked; he pushed himself further up. His hand struggled, gripped, found his mouth. His lips moved, were flanged outward, searched. A pink tip of tongue appeared and licked. His head lifted, swaying. Then it happened. Quite by himself, he found his mother's nipple, gaped as though his life depended on it, and sucked as he obviously had never done before, intensely, rhythmically. Everyone around smiled, relieved or surprised.

"How do you feel?" a Western expert asked the mother, who understood a little English. She was pale and young, with a broad, Slavic face. She looked up and answered haltingly, hesitantly but firm: "Dis is de happiest day in my life!"

To prepare for hand-expression, pumping, or breastfeeding a baby with a weak suckling reflex:

- Find a comfortable, quiet place close to the baby, or get a photo of the baby or a piece of the baby's clothing.

- Drink something warm beforehand.

- Warm up the breast before expressing or pumping.

- Massage the whole breast slightly.

- Stimulate the letdown reflex for several minutes by rubbing, massaging, rolling, or pulling the nipple carefully, using clean fingers, preferably over thin clothing.

To hand-express milk:

- Put your fingers about 1.5 inches behind your nipple.

- Position your thumb on the top of your breast and your index finger under it.

- Press your fingers straight inward toward your chest wall.

- Then press your fingers together, well away from the nipple, and then toward it a bit.

- Use a press-and-release rhythm.

- When the milk starts to come, keep expressing from the same place, for as long as anything comes.

- Then move your fingers around the areola until it feels soft all around.

- Do not slide your fingers on the skin—dry them if wet.

How often and for how long?

- Try to express or pump a total of about two hours per day.

- Divide this into five or six times, or preferably even more.

- Stimulate your breasts a little extra now and then when you get a chance.

- Get plenty of rest, and try to get at least six hours of unbroken sleep at night.

If hand-expression or pumping is slow:

- Change from breast to breast several times.

- Hang your breasts forward and massage and shake them.

- Stimulate the opposite nipple while pumping.

- Try to pump or express both breasts simultaneously.

- Finish when no more milk appears.

If you are breastfeeding a premature baby:

- Sit comfortably, and use cushions; this is going to take time.

- Hold the baby's body under your arm with the baby's head in your hand, or lie down comfortably, front-to-front with the baby.

- Let the baby lie calmly in peace; do not stress the baby.

- Prepare your breast and follow all previous advice for starting to breastfeed.

- Tempt your baby with a few drops of milk on the baby's lips.

- Allow pauses in the sucking; let the baby control the pace.

- The smaller the baby, the more frequently milk will be needed.

- If little seems to be happening, rub the baby's palms lightly as the baby sucks.

- Stimulate the opposite breast if the milk is slow in coming.

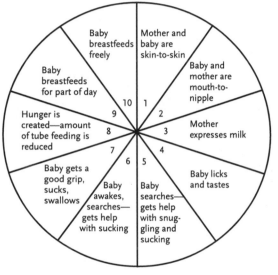

Breastfeeding of a premature baby must be done in stages—often with two steps forward and one step back.

The "Breastfeeding Wheel," based on an idea of B. Persson

Chapter 8

Postpartum: Blood, Sweat, Smiles, and Tears

"Thank you for what you said to me at the clinic," wrote Sally, "about going home to bed and staying there for a few days. I never thought I would feel so worn out. I wish I had known more about the postpartum period. I wasn't able to think about anything but the birth itself."

Midwives and others who teach Lamaze classes say the same: "It is almost impossible to get pregnant women to look beyond the birth. It's like a mountain on the horizon that blocks the view." This is a shame. Your body usually knows intuitively how to cope with childbirth. It is afterward that you really need information—especially these days, when, statistically, few have ever looked after younger brothers and sisters. The average family has few children, usually born a couple of years apart. Perhaps you don't have a lot of nieces and nephews, either. Your best chance is often with your friends' children. But being with them does not necessarily give you the experience you need.

Childbirth is an incredible challenge and a real test of strength for a woman's body. When the baby is born, you may think you have passed the winning post: "And now we all live happily ever after." Maybe. But even when everything goes well, the postpartum period is a very special time, and it can be helpful to know a little about it.

Bleeding

You lose a lot of blood during childbirth, and you will continue to bleed for some days. You will probably need to use sanitary napkins. Some women bleed for weeks, but most do so for only a few days. The blood gradually changes from bright red to brownish red to light pink. Finally, it becomes almost clear and watery before it dries up, usually after five to six weeks.

The womb continues to clear itself after pregnancy. Right after delivery, a large, bleeding surface remains where the placenta used to be. The muscle fibers in the womb normally contract quickly and cut off the blood vessels so that heavy bleeding stops. Putting the baby to the breast also helps this process. This stimulates the production of oxytocin, the hormone for milk production, which also causes the womb to contract effectively. The same hormone, artificially produced, is often used in the maternity ward.

Amy was still bleeding heavily when it was time for her to go home after four days. She was a little jealous of the others in her room, who were bleeding less than they would during a normal period. When the midwife checked Amy just before she left, she saw a little sliver of fetal membrane still hanging from the neck of her womb. This was carefully pulled out, without causing much discomfort for Amy. Thereafter, the womb contracted much more effectively, and the bleeding soon stopped. Like most other women, Amy found that her womb drained better when she had been lying on her stomach for a while. It was lovely to be able to lie like that again, with a pillow underneath her so that her breasts weren't squashed.

Things were a bit worse for Terry in the room next door. She had a lot of stomach pain, especially when her little boy was breastfeeding. Everybody told her that this was caused by postnatal contractions. She said that she had not felt this discomfort the last time she gave birth— but postnatal contractions become more common with each child. The more the womb has expanded, the harder it works to contract. Terry was given tablets to help relieve her pain. She was bleeding, however, and her womb did not appear to be contracting well. An ultrasound showed that a small part of the placenta was still inside her. First she was given medicine for a few days to get the womb to expel what was left in it, but that did not help. Then she was given a short-term anesthetic while the womb was cleaned out using surgical instruments.

Afterward, everything was fine. Perhaps we should have guessed what the trouble was, because Terry was producing little milk—even though she had produced plenty for her first child, and even though her new baby was sucking energetically. Occasionally, placental remains can slow the beginning of milk production. If the remaining part of the placenta continues to create pregnancy hormones, this limits milk production. It is exactly because of these hormones, that milk generally is not produced before childbirth, even though the breasts are ready for production during pregnancy.

The midwife or doctor usually discovers any remains of the placenta or the fetal membranes right after birth. It is not always possible to be certain that the womb is clear, however. Sometimes, in fact, the remaining placenta or membrane is not discovered until after the woman has returned home.

BLOOD COUNT AND IRON RESERVES

Blood transfusions are seldom administered these days unless blood count is very low. Even though all blood is tested as stringently as possible, blood transfusions are used only when there is a very good reason for doing so. This is mainly because of the fear of unknown viruses, contamination, sadly demonstrated in connection with AIDS. All blood used for transfusions today is free from the HIV virus, but the fact that some people have previously been infected through blood transfusions has been a shocking reminder to us all.

This means that you yourself must acquire the iron you need to create new blood corpuscles. You can do this by being very conscientious about your diet. Eat lots of dark green vegetables, fiber-rich foods, raisins, and beets. Because some people just can't eat enough to get their blood count up, however, it is a good idea to take iron tablets after childbirth as well. You may have done this also when you were pregnant. If so, you'll already know which iron tablets suit you best and don't upset your stomach.

Your blood volume increased by around 40 percent during pregnancy. Imagine an extra milk carton or two full of blood. A marvelous reserve, which means that you have something to go on. But the red blood corpuscles, which carry oxygen through the body, did not increase as much; your blood just became thinner. If your iron reserves are not high enough, you're going to need iron after birth like never before. You now must rebuild what you lost, because you probably lost more than you had in store. If you're deficient in blood, with a low blood count, you often get tired. And this comes on top of everything else that is making you tired.

Losing Fluid and Losing Weight

On average, most women gain 25 to 30 pounds during pregnancy. Anything from 18 to 40 pounds is considered completely normal. The baby, the placenta, amniotic fluid, and bleeding account for the many pounds, which generally disappear after childbirth.

You will also lose a lot of fluid after childbirth. In the course of the pregnancy, it is normal for the amount of fluid in your body to increase by 6 to 8 quarts. As a result of hormonal changes after childbirth, you excrete most of this through urine and sweat.

A few women return to their prepregnancy weight soon after birth. This shouldn't be a goal in itself. Of course, it's nice to be slim again—but most women also acquire a little layer of fat on the thighs and hips during pregnancy, which is the ideal situation. That fat is designed as a food reserve for the breastfeeding period. This layer of fat has been shown to begin disappearing for most women, without any extra effort, after three to four months of breastfeeding. In fact, breastfeeding is one of the best methods of getting rid of fat below the waist—and these are normally the extra pounds that get harder and harder to get rid of as the years go by.

Painful Wound from Cesarean Section?

The wound normally heals well following a cesarean section. Stitches rarely need to be removed. A cesarean section involves cutting and sewing through many layers, however, and moving around without painkillers is as a rule painful at first. Sometimes blood collects in the wound, or infection makes it extra painful. You may also develop a fever. The wound sometimes needs to be reopened slightly to drain out blood or pus. If a lot of blood or pus is present, or if it lies deep down, you may require another operation. If you have to cough—quite common following an anesthetic—this can cause pain. Try to press something, such as a rolled-up towel, against the dressing before you cough. This provides good support and stops the edges of the wound from moving so much, making the cough less painful. You will feel like staying in bed after a cesarean. You need a lot of rest, but beware of the risk of blood clots. If you are lying down for most of the day, move your feet a lot.

Do the Stitches Hurt?

Fortunately, you are not likely to be cut when you give birth. A few years back, all first-time mothers were normally cut. This was to avoid big tears, which could damage the mother in the long term and take longer to heal than cuts.

Now, most of those who help during childbirth see it differently. If the birth is going well and things are moving ahead gradually so that the tissue around the vaginal opening has plenty of time to stretch, even first-timers can often give birth without being cut. Some midwives use oil to make the opening even more slippery. Others heat the vaginal area with warm cloths. We know from athletics that warm tissue is particularly elastic and therefore less likely to tear.

Some women suffer from small tears, which require a few stitches. These rarely cause much discomfort. Sometimes it is necessary to cut for a number of reasons: the baby is particularly big; the tissue appears pale and taut and shows signs of tearing; the baby is in distress and needs to get out; suction cups or forceps are necessary. Sometimes large tears come as a surprise. Large tears may happen when the baby's head or shoulders are born quickly instead of sliding slowly out.

Lisa wanted to give birth as naturally as possible. She sat on a birthing stool leaning back against her husband. The midwife knelt in front of her. The birth went really well. Nonetheless, she suffered a large tear, which went right back to her anus. The doctor was called to sew it up. Lisa ended up with twenty-three stitches.

Every time Lisa rolled over, or walked a little, or went to the toilet, she felt incredible pain. She had dreamed of being the perfect new mother. She wanted to look after her baby herself and had planned to go home early. Instead, she staggered around bowlegged. Each step felt like a nightmare. She paled at the thought of her first bowel movement after giving birth. She just wanted to cry instead of chatting happily with all her visitors and boasting about her beautiful baby.

The following day was even worse, as is often the case. The stitches pulled because the tissues swelled and were irritated. There can be some infection, although this seldom happens. Painkilling pills, which also reduce the swelling, helped Lisa a little. She was advised to take a sitz bath with soft soap dissolved in the water. This was soothing and cleansing. A nice long shower with lukewarm to cool water also felt good.

Lisa had one stitch, which was a little too tight, removed before she left the hospital. Nonetheless, her tear was still painful. When she couldn't manage to sit in the bathtub at home, she used saltwater compresses.

"The stitches were most painful on the third day," she said. This is typical. "When I got home, I found a mirror and had a look. To be honest, I was horrified. It looked terrible. I thought I would never be normal again. Luckily, I had enough energy to laugh at myself, as I lay there with my legs apart, tending to that part of me, while milk ran from my breasts and the baby screamed. I said to myself that my colleagues should have seen me now. I was always so neat and well dressed. Anyway, my sense of humor improved quickly when the pain disappeared and I saw that my vaginal opening was actually beginning to look like it used to. And I am very glad the days of having stitches removed are over. The threads just disappeared by themselves eventually."

If you find it difficult to urinate after birth, find a time when you won't be disturbed. Turn on a tap. Stroke your finger upward along the inside of your thigh. Tap gently on your bladder. Read a magazine and think about something else. A soft plastic catheter inserted into the urinary tract is sometimes necessary to help you urinate in the beginning.

The vagina has an incredible ability to heal and return to normal after childbirth. It often takes just a few days. But even when a lot of stitches have been necessary, eventually it will look much as it did before the birth, thank goodness!

Sometimes, however, vaginal problems occur after childbirth, perhaps as the result of a tear that has not healed nicely and has left the vaginal opening a bit too wide. The main rule is not to do anything about this during the first six months, because the body continues to repair itself long after delivery. Even if it doesn't manage to repair perfectly, it is common to wait until a woman has given birth to all the children she wants before a repair is made.

Some people may have problems containing urine, air, or feces after childbirth. These are usually transitory problems. It sometimes seems a bit difficult to get the vaginal muscles to contract or release at will. Normally, however, these problems clear up on their own. In the end, you will get your muscles working again and can begin to tighten them and get them to react according to your will. Don't worry if this takes time. If the anal sphincter has suffered long-term injury, this can be operated on later.

Hemorrhoids: A Common Postpartum Problem

A lot of women get hemorrhoids—varicose veins around the anus—during pregnancy. This is the result of the increasing pressure in the abdominal cavity, which causes the membranes to swell. When the baby is ready to be born and you are pressing harder than ever before in your life, your hemorrhoids will probably become worse or may appear for the first time. After childbirth, you'll find relief in getting the swollen hemorrhoids—which may lie like a wreath around the anus—to drain and contract. Ideally, your midwife will see that this is done. A cold cloth pressed against the hemorrhoids for a while can help. Pushing the hemorrhoids into the anal sphincter also helps, although this is not always easy to do after childbirth.

Many people suffer as Melanie did. The small hemorrhoids she had during pregnancy now felt like a bunch of grapes after the delivery, she maintained. They just became more and more painful. Two days after she had given birth, the midwife in the maternity ward asked me to check them because she thought they looked so bad. Melanie's second phase of labor, when she had pushed the baby out, had been exhausting, lasting more than one hour. She had done her best and had produced a big, beautiful baby. But she had also acquired a ring of hemorrhoids. Someone had given her a topical ointment, but it hadn't helped much.

In this case, good advice was precious. The longer the hemorrhoids remained filled and on the outside of the anal opening, the greater the risk that the blood in them would coagulate, making them even harder to drain and more painful. Draining and pushing them back inside, past the anal sphincter, was necessary. Melanie hardly dared to touch them. She just lay there on her side with her legs tucked up under her, hardly able to walk because of the pain.

We tried a special remedy that helps most people in this situation. First Melanie had to raise up her bottom; she got onto her knees and elbows. The hemorrhoids were then at the highest point of her body and would drain more easily. While she remained like that, we applied a local anesthetic ointment. Then we covered the painful area with a rubber glove filled with crushed ice, well covered with a thin cloth so it wouldn't be too uncomfortably cold. The same principle works here as for a swollen ankle: keep the area elevated and put cold pressure on it. Melanie remained like that for twenty minutes while listening to the radio. Then her arms got tired, and somebody put some big cushions under her stomach so she could maintain the position while lying down.

After a while, the hemorrhoids had shrunk a little, and the local anesthetic had started to work. Then I put flat fingers on the hemorrhoids and pressed firmly while Melanie tried to relax her anal sphincter. First the hemorrhoids drained a bit more, and then we gradually began to reach our goal: they slipped back inside the anal opening. Now nothing prevented the venous blood from draining completely. In a few places, the blood had begun to coagulate, but these no longer hurt once they were back inside. Afterward, Melanie remained in this position for a good while to ensure proper drainage. Finally, she lay down with her legs close together, and over the next few days, she was able to push the hemorrhoids back in as soon as they popped out.

You can do this form of first aid—or parts of it—at home by yourself. Don't be afraid to use your fingers to push the hemorrhoids into place. Use disposable gloves if you prefer or just wash your hands well afterward. Sometimes, if the hemorrhoids aren't too big and sore, a cool shower is all that is necessary to make them shrink. Another handy home remedy that a new mother taught me is to cut the fingers off a rubber glove, fill the fingers with water, knot them, and freeze them. These cool objects are perfectly designed to fit between the buttocks.

Your Digestion

Many pregnant women have constipation, which also contributes to hemorrhoids. Following childbirth, new mothers are often impatient to go to the toilet, but those who have stitches and a sore vaginal area dread the first bowel movement. It can be painful, especially if the feces are hard. Because of this, women who have large tears that have been sewn up are often given stool softeners to make the feces softer. Most women really don't need a stool softener, however. Remember, you probably did not eat much on the day you gave birth. Perhaps you had a bowel movement during labor, or you may have had an enema beforehand. Often, little bowel content is produced the following day.

Nonetheless, it's sensible to think about your digestion when choosing what to eat after childbirth because it can be a bit difficult to get going. This is also partly due to the sudden change of pressure inside your abdomen.

Eat and drink as much as you can manage. Choose buttermilk or yogurt rather than fresh milk, and pick whole grain bread over white bread. Multigrain breads with various seeds are best because they often contain a supply of linseed and bran. If the hospital does not offer these choices, ask visitors to bring you some, as well as raw carrots, fruits, and prunes. Drink a lot of water. If you are used to having a bowel movement at a specific time of the day, or after a cup of coffee, try to get back into that routine.

Often we women fail to respect signals from our bowels. We may know that we need to use the toilet, but we have to do something else first. Especially when you have a tiny baby. The urge may disappear, and that is too bad. Without the emptying reflex, it is impossible to push out any feces.

Pay attention to signals from your bowels. Find a quiet moment, perhaps with something to read, in the bathroom. It may help to squeeze the stitches together or to press firmly against painful areas while expelling the feces. Afterward, remember to push the hemorrhoids back in again if they have popped out.

PELVIC AND BACK PAIN

While you were pregnant, your ovaries produced the hormone relaxin. This affected the ligaments that connect the bones of your pelvis, actually allowing it to become more elastic and to give way a little when the baby was born. As your belly got bigger when you got heavier, your posture also changed, straining your back. Because of these factors, together with psychological and social stress factors, about one out of three pregnant women develop troublesome back and pelvic pains.

If you had such problems during your pregnancy, they may continue right after the delivery. But for most women, the pelvis will soon recover. The ligaments will strengthen, and your back will eventually adopt its normal curves again. Unfortunately, however, some women suffer from back and pelvic pain for quite a long time. We will discuss this again in chapter 20. It is probably a good idea to try and avoid all movements that cause pain for the time being.

"My Hair's Falling Out!"

Jenny was really in a panic when she called me three weeks after the birth of her baby and complained that she had lost a lot of hair. "My pillow is full of hair when I wake up in the morning. When I comb my hair, great handfuls fall out. What on Earth is going on? Should I stop breastfeeding?"

Of course she shouldn't. Hair loss after childbirth has nothing to do with breastfeeding. During pregnancy, hormones prevent the hair that you would normally lose each day from falling out. This is why many pregnant women have healthy, thick hair. Once the baby is born and the afterbirth has been delivered, the high levels of hormones that kept your hair in place for so long disappear. Thus, you quickly lose the hair you should have lost during the whole pregnancy. For some women, it may seem that they have lost an awful lot of hair, but the process is quite normal and ceases after time.

Complete Exhaustion: Awakening During the Night

It is easy to get the impression that the maternity ward is populated by zombies—distant, apathetic, exhausted people. You normally do not feel like that the first day after childbirth—at least not if things went well. You are still on a high with the adrenaline from the birth. Eventually exhaustion does set in for many women, however—a reaction to the hard, physical work of childbirth. It was a time of high energy consumption and little food, of getting used to the baby, of looking after and feeding the baby—and also a time of frequently awakening during the night.

Most women find it hard to be awakened by their baby at night—not just once, but often many times. Even if you and your baby are having a peaceful time, your roommates may be keeping you awake. After a few nights, though, most new mothers are woken only by their own baby's cry, at least if they have been with the baby virtually all the time and thus know the baby well.

Several Scandinavian studies show that mothers who leave their baby in the nursery are no less tired than those who keep their child with them at night and breastfeed them. So let us acknowledge one thing: having a new baby is incredibly tiring. As a result, most Norwegian maternity wards have introduced a siesta—or period of rest—at some time during the day, when everything should be as quiet as possible. No visits or telephone calls, no meals or activities. It is a time for just resting. Preferably with your baby close to you, but if it is unsettled, let the staff take charge for a bit while you rest. Close your eyes. Even if you are not used to sleeping during the day, you will often drop off and wake up refreshed.

The Fog of Breastfeeding

Some of the drowsiness that you may experience during breastfeeding is what Norwegians call the "fog of breastfeeding." As a result of the hormones produced during breastfeeding, the new mother becomes relaxed and sleepy. Research has even shown that women score slightly less well on intelligence tests just after childbirth than they do otherwise. Perhaps this is nature's way of telling you to stay peacefully with your baby, to be more occupied with your immediate surroundings than with the rest of the world.

But relax: the fog of breastfeeding is only temporary. After a few months, you will be extra lively and wide awake, according to the same research report. This happens just at the time when the baby starts to turn over, to move around, and to need attention in a different way than during the newborn period.

Enjoy plenty of rest after you have given birth. Practice sleeping when you can. And remember—as soon as breastfeeding is well under way, it will have a relaxing and calming effect for you and your baby.

Using Visitors for Debriefing

Watch as women arrive at visiting time. All are very interested in hearing about the birth. Furthermore, they are more than willing to talk, often all at the same time, about their own deliveries. Experiences are compared and exchanged. Everyone is enthusiastic and emotional. The new mother seldom tires of recounting, again and again, what has just happened to her.

This tendency seems so strong that I wonder if it is a mechanism for protection. Could the exchange be a form of what is often referred to as debriefing? This term is used, for example, in crisis counseling. People who have been involved in a dramatic event are encouraged to recount in detail everything that has happened and how they felt at the time. Perhaps this is the best way to prevent a painful childbirth from leaving bad long-term memories and creating a fear of childbirth. Perhaps it contributes to preventing even more serious problems. So talk away. Find somebody else who will listen if your husband has had enough. This is quite normal.

When dealing with painful stitches and other pain around the vagina:

- Keep the area clean (use a hand shower) and well ventilated.

- Ask a midwife or doctor whether tight stitches can be removed.

- Try a sitz bath for twenty minutes twice a day. Make a sitz bath (in a washing bowl) either by (1) dissolving 1 tablespoon of medicinal soft soap in warm water or (2) adding ordinary salt to water until the water tastes like tears.

- Apply a wet compress moistened with salt water.

- Use a little ointment on sore areas after your bath.

- Air-dry the sore area, and then try fanning yourself.

- Try painkillers that also reduce swelling.

When taking care of tender, external hemorrhoids:

- Cool them down so that they shrink.

- Try ointments and suppositories.

- Put your bottom in the air. Use a bag of crushed ice on hemorrhoids. Make sure the bag is not too cold; use a cloth or compress between the bag of ice and your skin. After about twenty minutes, push the hemorrhoids inside the anal sphincter.

- Sit as little as possible. It's better to walk, stand, or lie down.

- Eat green vegetables, foods rich in fiber, buttermilk, and linseed to help your digestion.

- Don't push too hard during a bowel movement; wait for a signal from your bowels.

CHAPTER 9

. . .

The Comforts of Home

Perhaps, like Nina, you have decided to remain at home to have your baby. Nina chose to give birth to her second child at home in her double bed. The birth of her first child had gone well at the hospital, quite gently, without medical intervention or pain relief. Now, she wanted to extend her experience. Nina was a nurse at that time, and intensely interested in childbirth. Today, she is a midwife.

I was reluctant when I was asked to attend. Reluctant because, in my job, both women and babies are sometimes injured or die during childbirth. This cannot always be avoided at hospitals, either, but it can be particularly difficult for both parents and for those helping if something goes wrong during a home delivery. (Childbirth is so safe in the developed world today, however, that the birth will probably go well no matter where it takes place. This is particularly true when the woman has given birth vaginally before and no known risk factors exist.)

So, faced with something of a conspiracy—"I found a willing midwife, and I am going to give birth at home anyway, but we would feel very safe if you could be there, too"—I said yes. I went off with a pair of forceps in my bag, just in case.

And I experienced all the beauty of a home delivery. Nina, who puttered around in her own safe environment, chattered and laughed and ate and even danced a little between contractions. She ended up in the bath when things were at their worst. She did get fed up, tired, and impatient, but eventually she gave birth, sitting on the edge of their double bed, leaning against George. The midwife knelt on the floor in front of them. Everything was fine.

There was no transfer to the maternity ward and no tiring journey home. The birth was celebrated in Nina's own bed. She and the little baby fell asleep together. Everything was familiar and safe. Help flooded in, but Nina was in good shape. She and George organized it all—and enjoyed being with their children.

Only a small percentage of women in the United States choose to give birth at home; the practice is much more common in other countries. The debate has been both for and against. Much is in favor of births taking place in a well-equipped hospital, with staff well qualified to tackle possible problems. But, as in Nina's case, much can also be said in favor of giving birth at home. I am not going to debate this here.

Going Home

Some women choose an ambulant birth, where they go home a few hours after the baby is born. Others go home after a day or two. Studies show that returning home shortly after giving birth works just as well as staying at the hospital for a longer period of time, as long as a system is in place for home visits from healthcare professionals who can check both mother and baby and help with any breastfeeding problems that arise. The family is also expected to get support and help from friends and family.

The length of stay in maternity wards has been shortened considerably in recent years. From the vacation of the old days, with a week or two in a maternity ward, most new mothers and babies now leave after three to five days if everything is going well. Unfortunately, increased care outside the hospital has not followed this trend.

If you go home very soon after childbirth, you may need to return to the hospital for a screening for Phenylketonuria (PKU), a blood test taken from the baby's heel. This is to check that the baby does not suffer from a rare illness that can lead to increasing mental impairment. When this condition is detected in the newborn, help is available, and the child can grow up completely normally.

Going home from the hospital can be a shock for some people. Perhaps you longed to be home while you were in the hospital. The maternity ward was tiring and noisy. Nonetheless, you were surrounded by experts there, even though they were busy.

A Hard-Learned Lesson

Let me share my own experience with you. I was fit, young, and sure that everything was going to go perfectly well when my first baby was born. I turned down an offer from my mother, in fact, who wanted to come help, and booked my summer with friends from the south who wanted to see the north of Norway while we were living there. I did my utmost to make everything nice and memorable for the others. But I forgot one of the most important rules of the postpartum period: if you don't look after yourself, you won't be able to look after your baby properly, either. I was tired, undernourished, and worried, and the baby cried a lot.

All species that feed their offspring use a lot of energy to do this. The hard work that birds do feeding their young corresponds to whole days of physical work for a human. Mammals that have just given birth spend a lot more time eating than they did before, as well as looking after their young.

"Experience is an expensive lesson, but the fool doesn't learn from anything else," wrote the teacher of one of our boys, who always had to test everything out for himself. The next time I came home from the hospital with a newborn baby, the fool had learned from experience. I had organized a nice, clean house, and the beds were freshly changed. Granny was at home baking bread, looking after the baby's big brother. The freezer was full of food that was easy to prepare. I had no other plans than to be a mother. It was wonderful.

Home to Bed?

As a result, I often say to pale, new mothers with dark rings under their eyes, just before they leave, "Go home to bed. Get up to go to the bathroom, but spend as much time as possible in bed with your baby, at least for the first few days. Let visitors wait. Or just see the people you really want to see. If possible, take everything you need with you in bed: something to eat, something to drink, napkins, and cups. Let other people deal with everything while you stay in bed and be waited on. At least start out like this. You can always increase your level of activity if you are full of verve, and if the baby is content and breast-feeding is going well." Still today, a friend of mine visits newborn babies and their mothers with a beautifully carved wooden box of Norwegian rich sour cream porridge, just as people did in the old days.

If you are lucky, you have a helpful husband who can deal with all practical things for the first few weeks. Read more about this in chapter 4. But not everyone is that lucky. Is there anyone else you can call on? Your mother? Your sister? Your aunt? A friend? This is often a time when you feel a particular need to be with other women. You may want someone to talk to about the physical phenomena that no man can experience, whether bleeding or breastfeeding or the pain of childbirth that you experienced.

GRANDPARENTS

Recently I was talking to the beaming grandfather of a new baby with a single mother. The grandfather had taken early retirement, while the grandmother still worked full time. "I drop around nearly every day, and I really enjoy it," the grandfather told me. "I do the washing up and the cleaning. I go shopping and take the baby out in the stroller if my daughter needs a rest or a bit of time to herself. Often we do something together, all three of us. This is a wonderful experience for me. I never did this when my own babies were small." Not only young men can change.

Nonetheless, usually grandmothers get most excited about having grandchildren and try to help as much as they can. In Elaine Morgan's amusing book about evolution entitled *The Descent of Woman,* she recounts a developmental, historical reason for this tendency: of all the mammals, only the human female lives for a long time after she herself has finished reproducing. Morgan presents a theory about how this benefited the survival of the species. As our ancestors developed over thousands of years, the human baby had to be born ever earlier and ever more helpless. This was because the human brain gradually became larger over the generations, needing an increasingly larger outlet in order to be born. But also, the female pelvis changed in an unfavorable direction during the same period. Because she started walking upright, her pelvis needed to be stabilized so she could keep her balance. It became more rigid with less ability to let a baby through. Thus, only small infants born early enough would survive birth, which meant that they were very vulnerable and helpless compared to the offspring of most animals. In families where there was an older woman who was no longer fertile, and thus

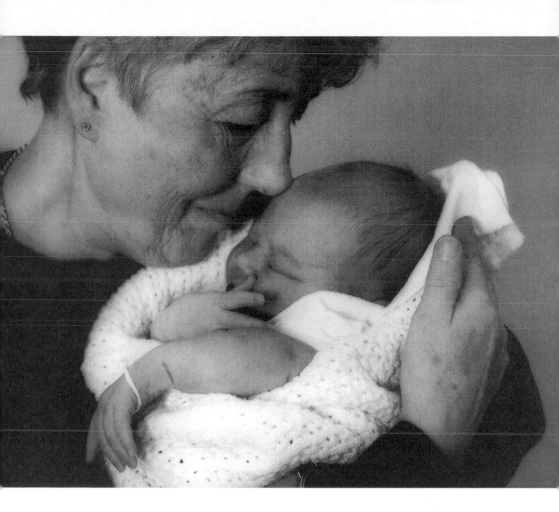

no longer busy with her own small children, things went better. Older women could use their experience and their energy to help the young women raise their children. A greater percentage of children from such families survived, and early menopause after many generations became the norm among women. No wonder most middle-aged women are gripped by an intense zeal and feelings they hardly understand themselves when they are expecting a grandchild!

THE CHANGING BODY

Many postnatal problems and difficulties with breastfeeding continue or first appear after you go home. Some mothers call me up then to ask, "What on Earth am I going to do? I'm producing skim milk! And my breasts are really soft. Am I going to lose the milk?" Of course not; that's how it's supposed to be. Mature milk looks different than the yellow colostrum first produced after childbirth. Swelling in the breasts and overproduction will disappear.

Pelvic pain often continues for a while. Try to make your life as pain-free as possible while your body tightens up and gets back to normal after the birth; avoid all painful movements.

Occasionally, the womb does not empty completely after birth. Joan was sitting in the bathtub at her home six days after she gave birth when she suddenly began to bleed profusely. Her husband was terrified; he stammered when he called me on the telephone at the maternity ward. He said Joan appeared to be swimming in blood, because there was some water in the bathtub as well as blood. We sent an ambulance, but by the time Joan got to the hospital, the bleeding had stopped. This is often the case. The bit left in her womb had become loose and was followed by bleeding. Then the womb could easily contract, and the bleeding stopped. Nature is clever at sorting things out. For safety's sake, though, it is sensible to contact the hospital or the doctor whenever heavy bleeding occurs.

"It's Driving Me Up the Wall!"

More and more young women have worked hard getting an education and career before they have children. They look forward to relaxing at home with just a sweet little baby to care for. Some plan to do things they have never had time for before.

Christie had a real shock. "I thought I would have plenty of time after a few weeks. I have always wanted to weave, and I also planned to paint and spruce up the apartment. I was going to read lots of books, which just lay there waiting for me.

"Daniel went back to work. The good life as a stay-at-home mom was about to begin. But the days just flew by. When Daniel came home, I was so tired. It seemed like I had been on the move the whole day, without any time to myself. No sooner had I finished changing and feeding the baby, had a bite to eat, and put a load of washing in than it started all over again. Sometimes I just had to carry or rock the baby for hours.

"It was tiring to go out, too. When I was finally ready, having got both myself and the baby dressed and the stroller out, he would poop in his diaper and scream loudly, and we had to go in again.

"I dreamed about meeting my husband at the door with a kiss, groomed and smelling wonderful. We would enjoy a delicious home-cooked meal that I had lovingly prepared, now and then looking in on our beautiful, sleeping baby.

"The reality was different. The house was a mess. Books lay unopened. Often I hadn't even started to make supper by the time Daniel got home. And my looks weren't anything to write home about, either. The clothes I had before I was pregnant still didn't fit, but no one was going to get me to wear my maternity clothes again. No matter what I did, I was spattered with drops of milk, pee, and poop.

"Daniel was usually very kind and helpful. But once when I was particularly tired, he asked me gently, 'What do you actually do all day?' I became furious. I wanted a divorce. I screamed and I cried. It took several months before there was a day that began to resemble my dream. Only now are we starting to enjoy ourselves."

Christie's story is typical. Remember that you will be constantly busy, without having anything to show for your effort in the short term. Remember, too, that in some ways you are worse off than both your own ancestors and women elsewhere in the world. You may have a washing machine and even a helpful husband, but you spend a lot of time alone with the baby just when you need company most. Mothers who are bored and isolated do not function as well as mothers who enjoy themselves.

If possible, it is sensible to prepare for the postpartum period before you give birth. Have plenty of suppers and bread in the freezer. Purchase some baby clothes in advance. Plan where you will change your baby's diapers. See to it that everything is in order and ready in that room.

Don't be too ambitious about having a clean house. Dust and clutter never killed anyone. Nonetheless, it is encouraging if your home looks fairly nice. You will wander around in a postpartum haze for a while. Allow yourself a period of time when it is all right to look a little disheveled and untidy. Comfort your husband by telling him it's going to get better eventually.

Single Mothers

Christie has a good husband in Daniel, and she has others who help. In contrast, Linda did not have such a large network of contacts. She is single, has moved a lot, enjoys her own company, and doesn't find making friends very easy. Since the birth of her baby, her needs have changed.

Linda described her experience: "I have always liked being on my own, but when I came home from the clinic with Ronnie, being alone drove me up the wall. I just wanted to be with somebody and to share the experience. I got terribly tired of the baby. I felt a bit calmer when I could hear voices, so I kept the TV on all day. I had to get out and see people. I was always going to the grocery store and talking to the employees. I even went to the library and borrowed books on child care and showed Ronnie off to the people behind the desk each week. When I told them that I felt I always needed to have the TV on, they showed me some audiobooks. Now I borrow romance novels, which I listen to when I'm bored. The best support I've found is at a group for single mothers organized by the well-baby clinic. It gives a much-needed opportunity for us to get together and talk about what it's like to be a single mother."

Linda has taken further steps to find out about special events and to meet people, and she has gradually created the network she needed. Several of the young, single mothers in her support group became her friends. They found fun things to do together, meeting at the mall or looking after each other's babies. Whether you are overwhelmed with offers of help or you have to work to find them, make use of them. Any way you look at it, being a new mother is difficult. It's easier if you don't have to do it all on your own.

Foreign Cultures

A young couple from Ethiopia told me the following: "In our country, the woman always returns to her childhood home well before the birth. She stays there until the end of her pregnancy, with help and support from her mother and other female relatives. She gives birth there and stays for several months after the child is born. Even if her own mother has passed away, she still returns to her childhood home, because we feel it is important that she feels safe in her surroundings.

The husband is there as much as he can and wants to be. If he lives far away, then he just visits." Not many modern women in the Western world might want to do this, but it is easy to understand the positive reasons for doing so.

A female doctor from India who was visiting the National Hospital in Oslo related a similar experience. "The woman goes home to her mother in the seventh or eighth month and stays there until long after the birth, often for six months. I myself went to my mother's after a cesarean section. It was lovely, because I can be myself at my mother's, but at my parents-in-law's, where we usually live, I always have to live up to certain expectations. I was only home for twenty days because we are modern people, my husband and I, and we would rather be together."

The Well-Baby Clinic and Pediatricians

After you come home with your new baby, you will have many days full of questions. Is the baby putting on weight? What are these red spots? When should my baby be vaccinated? Why is my baby screaming? When should my baby have vitamins? Is my baby developing correctly? Are we good parents?

This is why you should visit your local well-baby clinic or pediatrician. Some health centers send a health adviser to visit you at home, especially if this is your first baby—normally in the course of the first two weeks.

Some mothers find this visit a bit daunting. Your home isn't exactly how you like people to see it. Your baby, of course, has had an unsettled day. You hardly slept at all last night, and you are tired and messy. Perhaps the health adviser will think you are not a good mother.

Relax. The adviser sees this all the time. The purpose of the visit is to give you good advice and to detect any problems that perhaps you haven't seen yourself—for example, a too-perfect baby who sleeps nearly all the time and doesn't demand enough food.

The first checkup is usually after six weeks. Many prefer to come earlier, however, to weigh the baby or to discuss things they are worried about. The end of this chapter includes information about checkups and shots.

In addition to conducting standard baby checkups, the health center normally has plenty of useful information. Many health centers run groups. In these groups, mothers and possibly fathers with children of similar ages can get together and discuss topics. Many think this is a good idea and make new friends this way.

The health centers have useful brochures, and many lend out videos with titles such as *Breast Is Best* (see Resources, page 253), which answers a number of questions about breastfeeding. The health adviser can tell you where you can rent a breast pump and can give you information on postnatal exercises, physiotherapists who can help with pelvic problems, groups for parents with twins, and so on.

Advice on Breastfeeding

When you have left the hospital and good advice is hard to find, you can get assistance from a volunteer army of valiant foot soldiers: the mother-to-mother support groups, La Leche League. These are mothers who have themselves breastfed and who want to help others. They have regular meetings, read, learn, and have discussions before they take an examination and become recognized breastfeeding counselors. Visit their website at www.lalecheleague.org for more information.

Speaking to an experienced mother who knows a lot about breastfeeding can be incredibly helpful. Just remember that La Leche League mothers do not give advice about illness. Often they are working women with small children. Nonetheless, they freely give up their precious time in order to help you.

La Leche League always needs new recruits. Often those who struggle with breastfeeding themselves and who get help from La Leche League mothers later volunteer. You might want to consider joining some time in the future. It may also be possible to secure the aid of an International Board Certified Lactation Consultant. These highly trained professionals are often employed by maternity hospitals or pediatricians, or they may have their own practice where they offer consultations for a fee.

Help Is Available

Even if going home is difficult, and even if you don't have a good network of helpers, remember that you can still find help. In many places you are welcome to call the hospital in the first few days or weeks after you leave. If there is a health center nearby, it may be ready to help you even if you don't have an appointment.

About checkups and vaccinations:

- The baby needs checkups and vaccinations at set intervals. Check with your pediatrician or local well-baby clinic for their schedule.

- Most parents will want to make sure their babies have the following shots: diphtheria, tetanus, whooping cough, HIB, meningitis, polio, measles, mumps, and rubella.

CHAPTER 10

. . .

Infant Care

Your baby's small body is soft and delicate. The head wobbles; the arms and legs flail. You aren't sure what to do; you are worried that your baby might fall to pieces. You fear that you might injure your baby— or at least be so clumsy as to hurt it.

Don't worry so much. Newborn babies are robust. Nobody would think of holding an infant upside down or forcing it headfirst through a narrow tunnel. Yet your baby has just been through such an experience. The way out of your body was so narrow, in fact, that the plates of the baby's skull were pushed across each other in order for it to be born. Still, your baby survived—and most likely will be able to cope with a lot more shocks now that it is out in the world.

There is an old saying: "The first child is like the first pancake." Something to practice on. Obviously, you're going to be clumsy if you haven't looked after a newborn before. But the baby will help you. You will discover that your baby likes gentle movements, a constant temperature, and peaceful sounds. You will soon get the hang of it.

The most significant characteristic of the human baby is that the head is so heavy because it has to accommodate such a large brain. The spindly little neck, with its weak muscles, does not have the appropriate dimensions yet. As a result, you must be careful to support the baby's head when you move the body.

Otherwise, you do not need to worry about anything in particular in this respect, except to be careful about blows to the head. Never leave a baby lying on a changing table, because the baby might fall to the floor. If you know that you might be disturbed, change your baby on a rug on the floor, or move your newborn to the middle of your double bed before you answer the telephone or comfort your toddler.

Dressing and Undressing

Stan and Paula had clothing and diapers ready and waiting before they brought their baby home from the clinic. They had been given many useful items and had borrowed others. This is sensible because babies grow so quickly in the first six months that they don't manage to wear out all of their clothes. Stan and Paula figured they would mostly be at home anyway, with a washing machine and dryer, and didn't think they would need too many clothes.

Dressing the baby seemed very awkward in the beginning. Stan dressed his daughter for the first time in the nursery and felt that the nurses were watching every move he made and smiling condescendingly. The diaper was loose, and his baby's tiny arms and legs didn't want to go into the new baby suit. What's more, his little daughter screamed disloyally the whole time.

Remember that babies don't care how they look, as long as clothes cover their body. Most newborns hate to have their face covered. This important instinct has saved many babies from being smothered. The baby doesn't know whether something lying over the nose and mouth is dangerous. To avoid panic, think about how the baby was born. First, widen the neck of the garment into a circle. Then put the back of the baby's head through the opening before you gently pull the garment over the face.

Small fingers will curl up inside long sleeves. Fold the material back outside your own fingers and pull the baby's hand out through the opening before you pull the sleeve up over the arm. When you need to remove the shirt, take the arms out first before lifting the top over the baby's face. Have all the clothes lying unbuttoned and ready on the changing table, and put the baby on top in preparation for dressing. This way it's easy to see which part goes where.

Many people have difficulty knowing how much clothing to put on the baby, and this is an important issue. Newborns easily get cold, especially those who are thin. At the same time, they don't like getting too hot. Traditional all-in-one sleepsuits are comfortable for babies; add a blanket for sleeping. Check with a finger down the neck to feel that the baby is warm enough. Hands and feet are almost always a bit cooler, and this may make you think that the baby is chilly when that is not the case.

The Umbilical Cord

Stan had a special interest in his baby's umbilical cord because he had cut it. He thought the navel looked sore where the remains of the cord hung shriveled. However, it doesn't hurt when the stump of the umbilical cord falls off, normally in four to eight days.

The navel may be a bit moist or bleed a little. Clean it carefully with a piece of cotton dampened with boiled water or disinfectant. Contact health professionals only if the navel becomes very red and irritated. The baby may be bathed, even though the navel has not quite healed. The area will heal best, however, if kept as dry as possible between cleanings. The smallest newborn diapers usually come up to below the navel.

Choice of Diapers

Stan and Paula chose disposable diapers because they, like most other new parents, wanted things to be as easy as possible. Disposable diapers come in many different types, for boys and girls, for tiny babies and for bigger children. They are practical but expensive. Furthermore, the diapers from just one newborn turn into a mountain of rubbish. Large forests are required to make disposable diapers.

Some people choose to use traditional cloth diapers. These are a one-time purchase, but additional cost is incurred for electricity for washing and drying, laundry soap, and wear and tear on the washing machine—and, of course, extra work is involved. The cost of plastic pants and safety pins also add up. And if you choose to use a diaper service, the costs may actually end up higher than that of disposable diapers.

If your baby experiences a rash or soreness when using cloth diapers, the laundry soap may not have been completely rinsed out of them, or traces of urine or feces may have been left in the diaper. To avoid this, use the following method: Rinse dirty diapers in the toilet bowl before you put them in a bucket of cold water to soak. Have two buckets in different colors, one for wet-only diapers and one for feces-soiled diapers. Use a mild liquid soap without enzymes for washing. Wash diapers at 194°F with an extra rinse, without conditioner.

Bowel Movements

The baby's dark green bowel movements right after the birth are known as meconium. A baby who is breastfed rich colostrum will often have a bowel movement at almost every feeding. A full stomach triggers the reflex to empty the bowel, at least four times daily in the first few weeks, and then a minimum of once a day in the next month. A baby who has fewer bowel movements in the first few weeks and doesn't put on weight normally may not be getting quite enough food.

Bowel movements become gradually lighter in color during the first week. Breastfed babies have yellowish bowel movements with a freshly sour smell. A baby who is fed a cow's milk–based product normally has a light brown, foul-smelling bowel movement.

Stan noted, "I thought it was a bit disgusting changing a dirty diaper on a baby. But I was relieved that it didn't smell of shit. I am quite sensitive to horrible smells. After a while, I almost began to like the smell of the baby's yellow poop. Anyway, it didn't happen that often after the first month or so. Sometimes several days could go by between the dirty diapers, even though she was eating and growing as she should."

Then Stan had to go away for a few days. When he changed his daughter's diaper after he came home, he shouted to his partner, "What on Earth has happened? This smells completely different! Really horrible. Is she ill?"

What had happened was that the baby had had a few bottles of formula while Stan was away. His partner had missed him and had been a little depressed. She had had a lot of things to do and wanted to get out and get some fresh air with a few friends. Her mother had come to help with the baby, and a few bottles while she was baby-sitting seemed to be a good solution. But how could this make her bowel movements smell so bad?

Due to some of the carbohydrates in mother's milk, a particularly friendly sort of bacteria—*Lactobacillus bifidus*—thrives and develops in the gut of a breastfed baby. Large amounts of this benign bacteria fight off the more adult bowel bacteria—the bacteria that give bowel movements a nasty smell.

A breastfed baby will not get constipated. (Babies fed dairy milk–based products produce more solid feces and are more likely to develop constipation.) When the baby goes on to solids, the bowel movement becomes browner in color. If the transition to solids happens too quickly or with too much food, the bowel movement may become loose and slimy.

Changing Diapers

This task simply has to be done—every time the baby has a bowel movement or when the diaper is really wet. Initially, the baby will pee very often because of its small bladder capacity, producing at least five or six wet diapers per day, sometimes many more.

Have everything you need at hand: diapers, safety pins, diaper wraps, plastic pants, a bucket or bag for dirty diapers, paper towels or cotton wash clothes, wet wipes, water, soap, towels, and cream. Have extra cloths ready in case some are wet. If you live in a house with several stories, you may want to have diaper-changing equipment both upstairs and downstairs.

A good airing, without washing, may be all that your baby needs if there has been no bowel movement. Otherwise, just hold the baby's bottom under the running tap or wash it with water. Don't use soap unless it is really necessary, because soap dries out the skin's natural protection. Unperfumed, mild baby wipes or baby oil is also fine for cleaning.

More thorough cleaning will be needed after a bowel movement. Grasp the baby's feet between your fingers and lift up the bottom as necessary. Use cotton or soft toilet paper to wipe away the worst before washing. Make sure you don't miss any of the folds in the skin.

Remember that baby girls must be cleaned from front to back to avoid transferring feces to the vaginal and urinary openings. Do not try to clean inside the vagina, which is self-cleaning.

Don't pull the foreskin back when you wash a small boy's penis. This also has its own system for cleaning. Pulling back a tight foreskin can lead to small tears and subsequent scars, which may cause problems later. The little, wrinkled scrotum requires extra attention to get it clean.

Leave the baby lying with a bare bottom for a good while after you have removed a soiled diaper. This is good for the skin and is especially important when there is a tendency toward diaper rash. If you change the baby before feeding, wrap it in something absorbent or in a loose diaper to air, while feeding the infant at the same time.

Many babies urinate as they get cool when their diapers are taken off. You can save yet another diaper change if you wait for this to happen. When the skin is completely dry, use a good baby cream on a sore bottom. Otherwise, cream is not necessary.

FEEDING AND CHANGING AT NIGHT

When your baby needs attention at night, do as little as possible. Change the diaper only if there has been a bowel movement or if it is soaking wet. Keep the lights low, and don't talk much. Some people find it useful to feed and/or change the baby just before going to bed themselves; they enjoy picking up a sleeping baby for a "fill-up" just before turning in. Others find that the baby nevertheless wakes up at the same time at night whether bedtime was early or late; this extra feeding doesn't give any more peace at night. Find out what works best with your child. Most babies need breastfeeding several times during the night at the start. Read more about this in chapter 19.

BATHING

Bathing your baby isn't the rigmarole that many people think it is. Most babies love to be bathed, perhaps because it reminds them of what it was like when they were surrounded by amniotic fluid inside the womb. Some cannot stand being bathed, however. If this is the case for your baby, do not bathe her or him every day; just give an extra thorough washing once a day. Remember the folds behind the ears (never use cotton swabs in the ears), and clean the eyes with a bit of cotton— a new piece for each eye, outward and down toward the nose. Also clean the folds and wrinkles in the neck, the armpits, and the thighs. Some people prefer to clean these areas before bathing the baby.

It is quite OK to use a clean washing-up bowl or the kitchen sink as a bathtub in the beginning. Or you can buy a suitable tub or a baby bath. In any case, wash the baby's bottom following a bowel movement before putting her or him in the bath.

Stan was in charge of bathing his baby and invited us to watch the show when we came to visit. He was so proud that you would think this was the first baby in the world ever to have a bath. It was literally an event. He had everything carefully prepared: bath oil, mild baby soap, flannels, a big soft towel, diapers, and clean clothes. He was wearing a T-shirt and an apron with a toweling front. He put a little oil into the water to prevent the baby's skin from drying out.

Stan used his elbow to test the water. It should be a comfortable temperature, around 70°F. The room was nice and warm so that the baby wouldn't get cold when she came out of the bath. Stan grasped the baby's upper right arm with his right hand. He let the baby's head lie on his wrist, with his own forearm resting on the bottom so he wouldn't get a backache. He used a soft, thin wash cloth. Wet fingers are often just as good for washing in nooks and crannies. The baby lay quite still, with big, dark eyes; there was little doubt that this was enjoyable.

Stan patted his baby dry with a soft towel and let her lie naked for a while. He made bath time a peaceful, cozy time, with quiet chat and lots of physical contact. This little baby simply loved being stroked and patted.

After a few months, you can usually bathe the baby in a normal bathtub with a good rubber mat on the bottom. But remember that most babies at this age are very active, kicking and wriggling, so you may suddenly lose your grip. A clean adult can also get in the bath with the baby at this time. This creates a special feeling of intimacy and security. An inconsolable baby with colic can be calmed in this way as well. Shared baths can also help a baby who for one reason or another cannot—or will not—suck from the breast. In warm water, milk often runs freely, and feeding in the tub can be a wonderful new experience for your baby. Note, however, that the mother should probably not have a bath if she is bleeding.

THE SCALP

Sometimes a baby develops cradle cap on the scalp. This is not dangerous and does not irritate the baby. It often disappears with careful washing and use of a comb, if the baby has hair. If this doesn't work, you can buy a 1 percent salicylic Vaseline or oil from the drugstore. Tell the pharmacist what you need it for. Rub it into the scalp and let it remain overnight before you wash it out. A baby's hair normally does not need to be washed more than once a week. Use a very gentle soap that will not irritate the eyes.

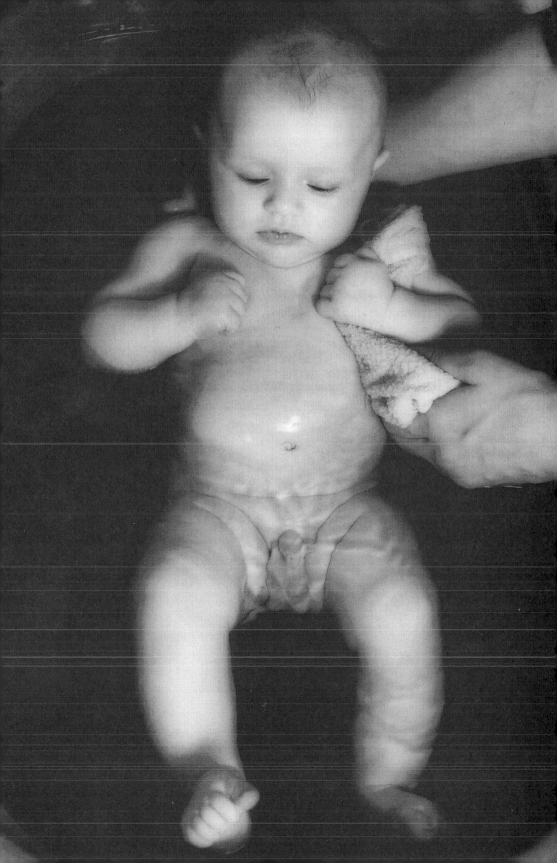

The Nails

In the beginning, babies usually have very soft nails. Still, babies can scratch themselves. At the hospital, small mittens may be used to prevent this. It is difficult to cut such tiny nails. The best way is to cut or bite off a little bit at the side and then pull off a flap of nail. Make sure not to tear the skin, as even small tears can become inflamed.

Diaper Rash

A baby who lies for a long time with a dirty or very wet diaper may develop a rash on the bottom and in the groin. Diaper rash will normally disappear with thorough cleaning, airing, good baby ointment, and frequent diaper changes. A little sunlight, for ten to fifteen minutes, can also help this type of rash. If it is too cold outside, you can sit inside the room so that the sun shines on the baby's bottom through an open window. Keep the rest of the baby dressed.

A persistent diaper rash may sometimes be caused by a fungal infection. You can use gentian violet or a fungal remedy to treat this. Talk to your health adviser or your doctor.

Red Spots

Some people think that red spots spoil the appearance of a newborn baby. It's not really surprising that the skin reacts to the transition from water to air—if this is the cause. "You should wait for three months if you want to have a pretty baby for the christening," one older nurse told me. She was right. For most babies, these rashes disappear after a few months and often earlier. They do not need treatment.

Fresh Air

Being outside is good for a baby and will help the newborn to sleep better. If the temperature is below 50°F or it is very hot, however, the newborn should not be taken outside. Instead, make sure the room is well aired. During the winter, the baby should be suitably dressed and, ideally, in a warm sleeping bag when outside. Daylight and sun are useful even in winter for the baby to obtain vitamin D through its skin.

In the summer, put the stroller in the shade, someplace where you can easily keep an eye on it. It may be sensible to fasten a net over the stroller to protect the baby from insects, birds, and cats.

If possible, put the stroller someplace where the baby can see a tree. At a very early age, babies are fascinated by branches and leaves that move. Some people maintain that this is particularly good for the child's development. In any case, the baby may lie awake for a long time, just watching.

If you live high up in an apartment building and don't have a balcony, a baby dressed in outdoor clothes can be put in the smallest room in the flat, with a large window open if possible.

In the Car

When transporting your baby by car, follow safety regulations. The baby should be in a car seat, which is fastened preferably with the baby facing away from the direction of travel. Rear-facing seats must not be placed on seats where inflatable air bags have been installed.

If you are going for a drive with your newborn baby on a cold winter's day, warm the car beforehand. If you're going for a long drive, take a changing bag and plenty of extra diapers and clothing. Many gas stations have baby-changing areas. Don't drive for too long at a time. Many babies really enjoy being in the car. Some even appear to go into a trance. Although the baby may appear to be sleeping peacefully, do not leave a longer break than normal between feedings.

Recommended baby clothes for when you're just starting out— better too large than too small:

- Six short-sleeved T-shirts and six pairs of pants (or all-in-one T-shirts and pants).

- Six long-sleeved T-shirts and six day/night clothes.

- Two pairs each of socks and mittens.

- Two caps.

- Two jackets.

- Two cotton blankets.
- Twenty-four diapers and six pairs of plastic pants.

Have the following ready before you change a diaper:

- Clean diapers.
- Pins and diaper wraps or plastic pants if you're using cloth diapers.
- Bucket or bag for dirty diapers.
- Paper towels and wet wipes.
- Water, soap, and baby lotion.
- Clean clothes.

Chapter 11

Breast Milk as Food

Think about launching a new sort of baby food that is automatically adjusted to the baby's changing needs for growth and development. Success would be guaranteed! The producer would become filthy rich. But the idea would come too late. It has already been invented: breast milk.

Let us make one thing clear: human milk is the best food for a human baby. All mammals create milk that is perfect for their own offspring. Still, most children who have never been given a drop of breast milk also grow up fine and healthy, fortunately, even if they miss out on the particular advantages of breast milk.

FAT

"Breast milk makes clever children" was the headline of a Norwegian tabloid last year. This is obviously a gross exaggeration, but it has a grain of truth to it.

Most organs are completely formed when the baby is born and only continue to increase in size. Not so with the brain, which is far from completed. The formation of brain tissue requires lots of fat. The major nerves have sleeves of fat, and the cell walls need fatty acids. And what is the best source for these fatty acids? Exactly, the fat in breast milk. It contains many of the long-chain fatty acids from which we all benefit throughout our lives, but which we need most at the start.

Extensive research has been done regarding the need for fat from human milk with reference to premature babies. The outstanding British professor Alan Lucas and his colleagues have compared premature babies who were given breast milk to premature babies who

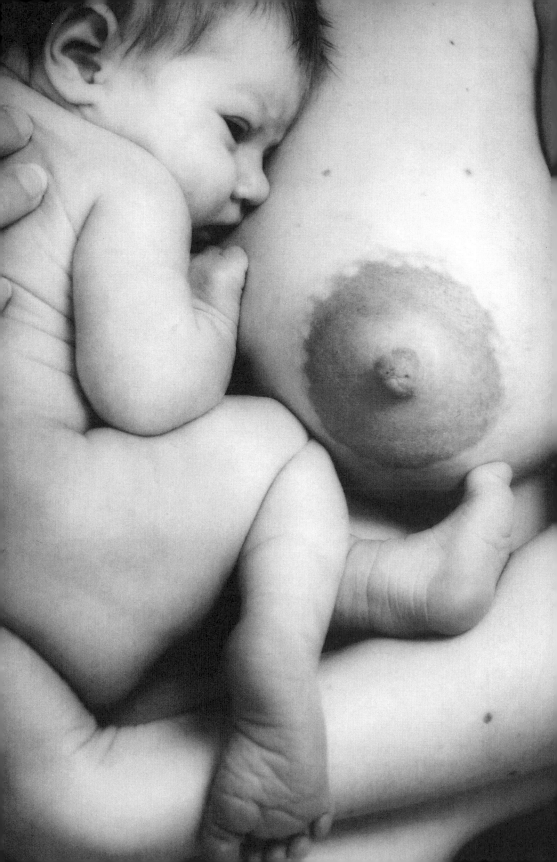

were not. The babies were given intelligence tests up to seven years of age. As in earlier studies, researchers found that breastfed babies did better on such tests than did babies who were not breastfed.

But Lucas knew that things other than breast milk itself could cause this difference. As a group, for example, women who choose to breast-feed their babies have a higher level of education than those who do not breastfeed. They also have a slightly healthier lifestyle, smoke less, drink less alcohol, and eat a healthier diet. Breastfed babies could also get more skin and eye contact, with small talk during feedings and with more lulling and cuddling.

Then Lucas developed a research project that could never have been done in Norway because almost everyone there is determined to breastfeed. English mothers who wanted to breastfeed their pre-mature babies were divided into two groups with characteristics as similar as possible with regard to the things mentioned earlier. Those in the first group were allowed to breastfeed their babies directly. Babies in the second group received their mothers' pumped breast milk through a tube. During later testing, the researchers found an equally good intelligence quotient (IQ) among the two groups of babies who had been given breast milk, either through breastfeeding or in some other way. Something in the breast milk itself must have a beneficial effect on the brain.

Mothers in a third group were like the others with regard to edu-cation and lifestyle but did not wish to breastfeed. On average, the babies of these mothers scored 8.3 IQ points lower at the age of seven than did the premature babies who had been given breast milk.

If you haven't fed your baby breast milk, relax. These differences are minor. The average IQ is 100. For anyone within normal limits, it is more important how intelligence is used than the exact number of points in a single test. Such differences could play a role for those in the lower part of the normal range, however. In any case, this study demonstrates how the milk from our own species is absolutely perfect for the brain development of our offspring. Similar findings have emerged in other studies, but Lucas's research is among the most thor-ough.

Creating and adding "human" fatty acids to formula isn't easy, and producing substitutes is expensive. These fatty acids are not made the same as their human counterparts are and therefore perhaps do not have the same effect. Finally, should manufacturers manage to make a satisfactory substitute, the worry is that the fat will go rancid in the packs on the store shelves after a while, and perhaps do more harm than good. Formula with added fatty acids now on the market have additives to prevent them from going rancid, but little documentation currently exists on the use of these formulas.

Breast milk, in contrast, is always fresh, straight from the producer. You avoid additional expense and the risk of contamination. The milk is served clean and at the right temperature. Its delicate packaging is also greatly appreciated. It is environmentally friendly, is always ready for reuse, and produces no waste.

Several studies have also shown that vision develops a bit better in premature babies given breast milk. Again, the fat is believed to be important, perhaps in combination with growth factors and other substances in the breast milk.

Studies of full-term babies point in the same direction. Some have also shown that breastfeeding for a long time gives better results than breastfeeding for a short period of time. The brain and the fat covering the large nerves continue to develop in the baby for the first few years.

As already established, fat is an important constituent of breast milk. On average, it provides half the calories. This benevolent fat is finely distributed in very small drops, and the baby benefits from practically all of it. This is perhaps the explanation for additional exciting results from the previously mentioned researcher Lucas. He has shown that full-term babies who for one reason or another have gone hungry in the womb put on weight faster when fed breast milk than when fed anything else.

These babies, small for their age when born, are thin, with loose skin and without the usual layers of fat. Because we want them to grow well, and because they constitute a risk group, these babies often receive formula supplements at birth. This may be necessary, because they can easily develop low blood sugar levels while waiting for their mother's milk to come in properly. At the same time, these babies must suck a lot on their mother's breast and get every single drop offered. One problem with supplementation is that the baby can lose motivation to suckle. Then, when the breast milk does come in later, the mother already feels that she is a failure, and the whole breastfeeding process is threatened. So take note: supplement if necessary, but not too much!

Do you think it sounds strange that there is so much fat in breast milk? Do you think the milk looks like water or skim milk? It isn't easy to predict the exact composition of breast milk because it changes all the time, in pace with the baby's needs.

Elisabeth has given me many a good laugh. She consulted me all through her pregnancy, and her descriptions were generally unusually graphic. "I thought that the colostrum was quite disgusting to look at, at first, almost like pus. But then someone said that I should think of it as delicious custard, which was nicer to give my little girl," she told me.

This first milk, colostrum, is beneficial and important. It at first acts like a laxative so that the baby will get rid of the meconium—the first feces—that has been in the bowel for a long time. You can read more about the marvelous properties of colostrum in chapter 12.

After the milk changes, it looks more normal. Elisabeth was convinced: "Well, there isn't much fat in my milk anyway! The drops I squeeze out now are almost clear." She felt reassured to know that the fat content varies through the day and during a feeding. The fat content usually increases toward the end of the meal. "Really clever," Elisabeth commented. "When I'm both hungry and thirsty, I too want a drink first before I start on the food."

The proportion of fat also generally increases during the day. This suited Elisabeth because she usually had less milk in the evenings. "Then I can just sit and console myself that she's drinking full cream from my lean boobs while I'm watching the evening news," she said happily. "The fact is that she usually falls asleep with a big fat smile, even if I didn't think that she'd had very much." This is typical. The fat releases substances that make the baby sleepy. Can you think of anyone more satisfied than a baby going to sleep, head askew and mouth half open, with the last drop of milk glistening on a lower lip?

The amount of fat in the milk decreases slightly if you breastfeed for many months, well beyond the time when the baby has started on other food. This is clever because then the baby can and should get calories from many different sources. However, only mother's milk gives the specific antibodies that protect against disease—substances that the baby makes good use of for a long time yet.

A small tip: Do you have a baby who cannot breastfeed directly, but for whom you are nevertheless producing milk? Perhaps because of illness or prematurity? Do you have more milk than the baby takes? Then it may be beneficial to express the foremilk and aftermilk in different portions and make sure that the baby at least gets the fat aftermilk if putting on extra weight is necessary.

Sugar and Other Carbohydrates

Remember that the fetus received nutrition constantly, day and night, and presumably never felt hungry. The mother's blood continuously fed the baby. Then this nourishment was suddenly cut off. Hours now pass between the baby's feedings. What is most urgent, then, when she eventually gets fed? When the baby is perhaps weak with low blood sugar, feeling starved?

First the baby needs something that will quickly increase its blood sugar level. It's good to know that breast milk always has plenty of sugar in it, and that the first milk the breast delivers during a feeding contains even higher levels. The baby's stomach and bowel absorb the milk sugar in an instant, which gives the baby the strength to suckle further and get everything the milk has to offer. But starting out, the baby needs sugar most. Clever, isn't it?

Breast milk contains many different kinds of sugar and carbohydrates. The milk sugar, lactose, is the most important for nourishment. Among other things, it contributes to the baby's ability to easily absorb the calcium in milk. Other kinds of sugar have other interesting properties. They help a beneficial bacteria—*Lactobacillus bifidus*—flourish in the baby's bowel, for example. These knock out other bacteria and contribute to easy digestion and the pleasant smell of a breastfed baby's feces.

Protein as Nourishment

Full-term babies make perfect use of the protein in breast milk. Bigger quantities of protein become a load. Cow's milk contains far too much protein for small human babies. That's why people learned in the old days to dilute cow's milk with a lot of water when feeding it to babies. But cow's milk contains too little sugar, so this had to be added. In this way, the efforts to artificially achieve nourishment that resembles breast milk continued, eventually resulting in the present-day formula.

Premature babies need extra protein. Nature is wisely organized so that women who give birth prematurely create milk with more protein. Premature babies should therefore be given milk from their own mothers as soon as possible. It is better suited to their needs than mature human milk from a milk bank if available.

Babies born very prematurely would normally have been nourished through their mother's blood for a long time. As a rule, they therefore require extra supplements of protein, among other things.

Iron, Other Minerals, and Trace Elements

William was two months old. His grandmother thought that he looked a bit pale and sickly; she felt that he needed more iron than he was getting from his mother's milk. When her children had been babies, they had been given solid food from eight weeks old. Also, she had read that breast milk didn't contain much iron. Perhaps a breast milk supplement enriched with iron would be better?

William's mother grew uncertain and sought advice. William was a fine young baby with a good weight gain; he was lively and content, even if he really was a bit pale. A blood test revealed an excellent blood count for a baby—lower than in adults and bigger children, as it should be. The test result did not come as any surprise to the doctor. In the first six months, breast milk is generally the very best protection against iron deficiency or anemia.

No type of milk contains much iron. The difference is that the iron in breast milk is specially made for the small human baby. William's mother marched proudly home from her doctor equipped with figures to convince her mother: "William's bowel is able to take up only around 4 percent of the iron in formula and 10 percent of that in cow's milk. But he can use up to 50 percent of the iron from my milk!" She continued happily with exclusive breastfeeding until William was six months old. Then it was time for the first little bit of solid food.

Premature babies, who do not have a fully developed bowel and have not built up any iron reserve, must sometimes be given extra supplements. Babies must not get too much iron, however, as it provides a base for the growth of harmful bacteria in the baby's bowel. As so often, meddling with nature proves to have unforeseen and often unhealthy effects.

Breast milk contains many minerals that the baby needs, and all in the right quantities. Zinc, for example, is necessary for humans. It is good for the skin, counteracts rashes, helps wounds heal more easily, and promotes growth in general. Zinc in cow's milk is bound to large molecules that are difficult for the baby's bowel to absorb. After all, that milk is made for a calf's stomach. The zinc in breast milk, in contrast, comes in small molecules that the human baby can easily absorb. Breast milk may have a good effect on some skin problems of artificially fed babies.

There is no mineral or trace element essential to a baby that breast milk does not contain in the right quantity. Eat a healthy diet and cuddle up with your baby. If possible, feed nothing but breast milk for the first four to six months.

VITAMINS

Breast milk largely contains all the vitamins that babies need for the first six months, with the possible exception of vitamin D, the fish oil vitamin. Everyone needs this vitamin for the bones to absorb calcium. The most common way for people throughout the world to get vitamin D is through sunlight. A little sun on parts of the skin for an hour a few times a week is enough. The problem arises in countries with long periods without much sun. Those of us who live in such parts of the world therefore have a pale skin that produces this vitamin extra quickly with just a little sun. We also have a tradition of drinking cod liver oil or of getting vitamin D in other ways at the darkest times of the year.

Not all of those who immigrate to such regions have this tradition. Ishmael and Begum were proud of their firstborn baby, a little boy. But when the boy was one year old, he was quite bowlegged and his rib cage slightly deformed. He had developed rickets. His skeleton was soft and contained too little calcium. What was the reason?

Begum had fed him as she would have done back home in Pakistan. With more than enough sunlight there year-round, extra vitamin D would not have been needed. The baby also had dark skin and therefore had more difficulty producing the vitamin himself from what little sun was available. He spent very little time outdoors because Begum found it was too cold. Language problems made communication with the health center difficult, so no cod liver oil had been given.

But what about people with fair skin? Must they be given vitamin D? Vitamin D is recommended for everyone in Norway from four weeks of age. Mothers who think that cod liver oil is messy often question the necessity, however. Then I permit myself to give individual advice. If you make sure that your baby is outdoors a lot and you yourself get plenty of vitamin D, then you will be OK. The quantity in the breast milk will increase when you take cod liver oil yourself instead of giving it to the baby. The same thing happens with the beneficial fatty acids.

Another vitamin that is heatedly debated among professionals is vitamin K. Very occasionally coagulation—or clotting of the blood—does not work as well as it should in newborn babies. Eventually vitamin K is made in the baby's bowel and contributes to the system of coagulation. In some places, newborns are given vitamin K routinely, either as drops or through an injection to prevent serious bleeding.

By trying to correct one thing, however, we may inadvertently cause something else unforeseen. Injections of vitamin K have been associated with a slightly increased risk of cancer later in life. Perhaps what we gain in one area we lose in another. In any case, parents do not need to be concerned with vitamin K. The health service must balance possible advantages and disadvantages based on the knowledge that exists at any time and do what they think best. Parents are free to protest against artificial supplements, of course.

Otherwise, breast milk contains everything the baby needs, including vitamins and trace elements. Wait before giving your baby orange juice. Drink it yourself. The baby will get enough vitamin C through your milk and will avoid the direct addition of foreign substances, which are thought possibly to provoke allergies.

FLUID

The old expression "There is a lot of food in a good drink" could have been coined about breast milk. But what about the baby's thirst on hot summer days? Or when it is running a fever?

Many people believe that the breastfed baby needs extra fluid if it is hot. Studies from the tropics have shown that babies, even during intense heat waves, maintain a normal fluid balance as long as they get the usual amount of breast milk. Don't mess around with the fine balance in the baby's bowel by giving water or anything else. These fluids serve no purpose and may cause harm. "Intoxication" from too much water has actually been reported in medical literature.

When breastfeeding is well established, breastfed babies grow especially quickly. The breast milk helps the baby's bowel mature so that the changeover from obtaining nourishment through the umbilical cord to obtaining it through the mouth goes well. Breast milk is so easily digestible that the nutrients are absorbed quickly. This is one reason for the need to feed breastfed babies more often than bottle-fed babies.

After about three months, however, an exclusively breastfed baby is on average a bit slimmer than a supplement-fed baby. The World Health Organization is currently working to create a growth curve that will show the "gold standard" for exclusively breastfed babies that will not compare them with babies fed in other ways. Under the current system, many babies are diagnosed as being underweight, while excess weight is recorded too late. In our part of the world, where obesity is a major national health problem—even for children—we need to remember that bigger is not necessarily better. A new major German study shows that children who were formula-fed as babies had a 4.5 percent risk of being overweight upon starting school, whereas those who had been breastfed had a much lower risk. The longer the breastfeeding, the lower the risk of later obesity.

Breast milk contains what the baby needs:

- Fat and—not least important—long-chained fatty acids.

- Sugar and other carbohydrates.

- Protein, albumen, enzymes.

- Iron, other minerals, trace elements.

- Water, salts, calcium.

- Vitamins (vitamin D supplements may be needed).

- Enough fluid even on hot days.

CHAPTER 12

. . .

Breast Milk as Medicine

"There is a reason for everything in nature."—*Aristotle*

I sit and leaf through the daily paper. As usual, there are big headlines. One story today is about vaccines: some have side effects; others don't really help. We must remember, though, that vaccination has saved countless babies and will continue to do so.

Think about what would happen if a new vaccine appeared that could save the lives of more than one million babies every year. This vaccine would have absolutely no side effects and would be incredibly cheap to produce. No refrigerators would be needed for storage or syringes for administration. Such a vaccine would become enormously popular and in instant demand for distribution throughout the world.

Yes, you may have already guessed correctly; I am talking about breast milk. The content of the preceding paragraph comes from an editorial piece published in *The Lancet,* one of the world's foremost medical journals. An enormous amount of research about breast milk is being carried out today. We who work with breastfeeding can barely keep up. In this chapter, I can include only a little of what we know today.

Doctors have known for a long time that breastfed babies are sick less often than bottle-fed babies are. Many have believed that this is largely because of the risk of poor hygiene with supplemental feeding. Research has gradually shown, however, that breast milk actively helps the baby to avoid illness.

ANTIBODIES

Think about little Frances. While she lay in her mother's womb, not only was she nourished, but antibodies were transferred to her from her mother. These antibodies have a limited life span, however, and not all types of antibodies crossed over to Frances. The placenta is very fussy about the size of what it lets through; it is like a fine-meshed wire fence through which a mouse—but not a cat—can pass.

What Frances needs most immediately after birth are the antibodies called immunoglobin A, or IgA. She had little of these antibodies as a fetus. Then she lay sterile in amniotic fluid, not threatened by infections. Now she needs to protect her mucous membranes. Although nearly invisible, mucous membranes line many of our body passages and cavities and serve an important function.

I once heard a world-famous professor of immunology ask members of his audience how big they think their skin surface is. The answer? About 2 square yards for an adult man. Then he asked how big the mucous membrane surface is including the digestive and respiratory systems. Wild guesses were made. Some took a strong stand and suggested 12 square yards. Wrong. The mucous membrane is around 480 square yards, large enough to cover nearly two tennis courts.

Newborn baby Frances's mucous membranes take up less surface area than do an adult's, but even so, they constitute a battleground open to infections. Only a single cell layer separates her from potentially life-threatening bacteria. This is why it is so good that breast milk contains large quantities of human-specific IgA right from the first drop. IgA clings to the mucous membrane throughout the long digestive tract and sort of coats its inside. Sticking there like flypaper, IgA deals with bacteria and viruses as they come in.

Antibodies can be vital, especially at first, because the baby is born with a weak immune system. The protection given through the placenta gradually lessens. Breast milk protects the baby through the transitional period of slowly building up an immune system. In fact, the baby's defense against infection is not fully developed until several years after birth. For this reason, the World Health Organization and UNICEF recommend breastfeeding for at least two years, while in the U.S. and in Norway, the official recommendation is for "at least the first year."

Milk from Mother Is Best

The ideal situation for Frances is to receive milk from her own mother. All breast milk contains IgA and works well. But the mother's IgA is specifically directed against harmful microorganisms in exactly this

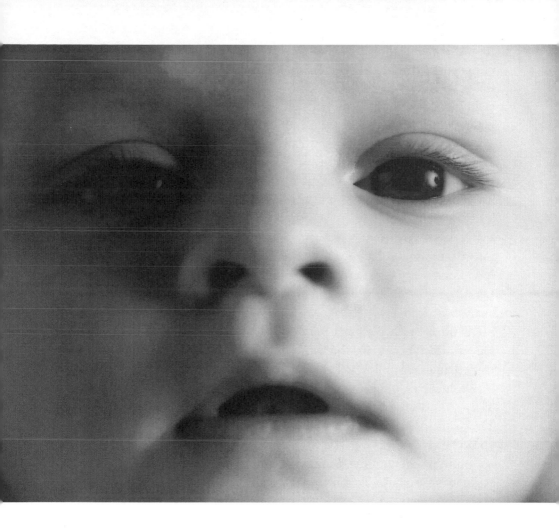

family's environment. In fact, it is adjusted so craftily that the mother transfers to Frances antibodies against most of what her own immune system has been exposed to throughout her comparatively long life. This protects Frances against all the intestinal infections her mother has had and probably against respiratory tract infections and other infections, too.

An exciting system called *homing* (named after the instinct of pigeons to always fly home from wherever they are released) has been demonstrated as an internal protective device among humans. At seven years old, for example, Frances's mother had a stomach infection, with vomiting and diarrhea. Her immune system then started to produce a special antibody exactly fitted to this bacteria, like a key to a lock. The mold remained, and when she was later exposed to the same infection, her immune cells quickly remembered how to produce this antibody so that she did not get very sick. This is the same principle behind vaccination: memory cells are trained to quickly produce specific antibodies.

These memory cells eventually settle down in the milk glands and produce large quantities of IgA for the baby, who needs it so much. If the same communicable disease bacteria infect Frances in her first years of life, she will have a mild reaction to them and will soon recover.

Because of homing, breastfed babies are far less vulnerable to infectious diseases than are bottle-fed babies. Cow's milk also contains IgA, but at only one-tenth of the concentration found in breast milk. Cow IgA is wonderful for calves but does not protect human babies against infection.

Human milk contains much more IgA than does the mother's blood, which nourished the baby while it lay sterile in the womb—10 to 100 times more IgA, in fact. The first milk, colostrum, contains even more. In developing countries, this is often a matter of life and death. There, bottle-fed babies frequently die from diarrhea or pneumonia. This is the basis for the calculation that more than one million babies could be saved every year through exclusive breastfeeding for the first six months and continued breastfeeding for two years. Life can be at stake in industrialized countries as well. Blood poisoning, menin-gitis, and diarrhea still kill our babies, but they occur less frequently among breastfed infants.

An interesting tale from a large Norwegian University hospital illustrates the importance of the specific antibodies. A serious intestinal epidemic occurred in the pediatric ward. Several children were gravely ill with diarrhea, and two died. Finally, the dangerous bacteria causing it was discovered. That particular bacteria is exceedingly rare in Norway but is more common in other parts of the world. Then someone got the idea to search Oslo for breastfeeding mothers from countries where this bacteria is more common. Several of those found had antibodies against this bacteria in their milk because they had themselves been exposed to it as children in their native countries. When the Norwegian babies were given milk donated by these mothers, the epidemic passed, and all recovered.

A common home remedy for an ill baby is to drip a few drops of breast milk into the baby's stuffed-up nose or inflamed eyes. Many women continue to do this and maintain that it helps, and the practice may have some rationale to it. Both nose and eyes are covered with mucous membrane, which may benefit from the IgA in breast milk. It has been demonstrated that when the baby suckles, the throat is "showered" with antibodies every time it swallows. This is one of the reasons that breastfed babies hardly ever come down with infections of the middle ear, which is connected to the throat. All types of respiratory illnesses, such as colds, bronchitis, and pneumonia are also much rarer in breastfed babies compared to those that are formula fed.

Breast milk contains many antibodies other than IgA, but this is the most important and can serve as an example. Because IgA attacks only harmful bacteria, all beneficial bacteria in the body remain undamaged and useful. In this way, breast milk is different than antibiotics, which also clear out the bacteria we need.

WHITE BLOOD CELLS IN BREAST MILK: THE BABY'S BODYGUARD

Breast milk is sometimes called white blood because it contains so many white blood cells. These cells are the body's police. The most common of them eat harmful microorganisms and give signals to other cells to start up their defense systems. The biggest of them, the macrophages, not only eat microorganisms, but also emit a substance that dissolves the bacterial wall. And who can manage without skin? The craftiest of them become small antibody factories, or memory cells, ready to react. White blood cells of a certain type are even called killer cells. The exciting thing about these is that they behave differently in milk than in blood. If killer cells in the milk come into contact with the E. coli bacteria found in the bowel, they reproduce vigorously and make an enormous effort in the war against the E. coli. This is especially important because E. coli can be fatal to the baby.

OTHER HELPFUL INFECTION FIGHTERS

Other useful molecules present in abundance in breast milk also help protect the baby against infections. Some produce mucus, which surrounds the microbes and prevents them from doing damage. Others work more indirectly. Following are a few examples.

As mentioned, too much or too little iron can cause harm. Many dangerous bacteria grow and multiply extra vigorously if excess iron is left in the gut. One of these, for example, is the feared staphylococci, often called the hospital bacteria. However, the iron-binding protein in breast milk, lactoferrin, binds the iron so that the bacteria cannot get hold of it. For this reason, among many others, unhealthy bacteria do not flourish in breastfed babies.

The sugars in breast milk promote the growth of the benevolent bacteria *Lactobacillus bifidus,* which for one thing occupies the surface of the gut, displacing the harmful bacteria and halting their reproduction.

Breastfed babies also have some protection against chicken pox, an illness feared in babies. Even if the mother has not suffered from the illness herself and does not have any antibodies, some fatty acids in breast milk damage the membrane that surrounds the chicken pox virus and help render it harmless.

Interferon is one of the body's strongest virus fighters. Particularly high levels are found in colostrum, the baby's food at the exact time when it needs protection the most.

A mother who had heard my lecture on breast milk called me, slightly offended, and said, "My boy has caught a cold even though I'm breastfeeding. What do you say about that?" The answer is that even with breast milk, a baby will still be ill sometimes. Illness will occur less often and will not be as serious for the breastfed baby, however. Just like careful driving significantly reduces the risk of injury, an accident can still occur. Because this woman's son was given breast milk from the day he was born and will probably be given it for a long time, he has less risk for a number of infections than does a bottle-fed baby. This is true not only of the dangerous infections we have already mentioned, but also of the more common ones as well.

Breastfed babies as a group need a doctor less frequently and are admitted to hospitals less often than are bottle-fed babies. Breastfed babies suffer less from diarrhea, the common cold, pneumonia, asthma, ear inflammations, and urinary tract infections, a few of the common potential problems.

Necrotizing Enterocolitis in Premature Babies

I visited a major hospital in New Orleans a number of years ago. A researcher there paid to get hold of newborn puppies that would otherwise have died. She used them for research to try to solve the puzzle of the dangerous disease called necrotizing enterocolitis, or NEC, which kills many premature babies. NEC leads to gangrene in the gut, which more or less falls to pieces and, of course, causes peritonitis.

I told the scientist that we rarely see this unpleasant disease in Norway anymore. Practically all premature babies here are given breast milk. The researcher shrugged her shoulders and would hardly believe that the answer could be so simple. Let's hope that time and the publication of a series of scientific reports have by now convinced this researcher and the medical establishment so that the unwanted puppies in New Orleans fare better these days.

Research in this field is so solid today that even the biggest skeptics finally agree. Among 900 premature babies in England, each weighing less than 1,850 grams at birth, the risk of getting NEC was found to increase tenfold for the group not given breast milk. Other studies have found an even greater risk increase.

This probably involves several factors. For one, breast milk has positive effects in striking down infections and at the same time promotes the growth of good bacteria in the gut. For another, colostrum starts a rapid maturation process of the gut. This is one reason why a few milliliters of human breast milk is put regularly into the stomachs of even the tiniest premature babies in Norway throughout the day. This is even given to babies so small that they cannot actually digest anything much themselves. These babies need to be fed intravenously for a long time; remember that they should still be being fed through the umbilical cord. Even so, a little breast milk in the gut is useful.

Breastfeeding and Allergies

Sandra's husband was bothered by eczema. She herself had hay fever and a slight food allergy. Little Matthew took most after his father. As a one-year-old, the youngster was covered with itchy eczema. He scratched himself so much that he needed mittens tied on at night. Sandra and her husband tried all the remedies they could find— homeopathy, baths with oat bran or oil, moisturizing creams—but none helped. In fact, only strong medications helped—but the parents were unhappy about giving these to such a small child.

Sandra had breastfed her baby. Starting had been a bit problematic. He had been given a few bottles of formula by the staff in the maternity ward after birth. Sandra had also given him some formula at home. From three and a half months of age, he was given mushy food and, eventually, dinner. The amount of breast milk then fell so sharply that Sandra stopped breastfeeding when Matthew was six months old.

Sandra came to me because she was pregnant again. She wanted to do whatever she could to prevent her next baby from having the same problems. Should she avoid certain types of food? Should she breastfeed exclusively without anything else at all? If so, for how long?

The discussion has raged back and forth regarding allergies and infant feeding. Many people hoped that breast milk would provide total protection against allergies—but it doesn't. Allergies are partly inherited and partly triggered by the allergy-provoking substances to which we are exposed.

To date, a number of research reports show that breast milk gives partial protection against allergies. If a genetically susceptible individual was breastfed as a baby, allergy symptoms usually appear later and in a milder form. Particularly regarding eczema, breastfeeding has recently been shown to have a positive effect up to adulthood.

With regard to a special diet for the mother during pregnancy and breastfeeding, we are cautious about recommending this in general. In some badly affected families, however, a special diet may be worth trying. A baby may benefit if a mother avoids the types of food that she and/or the father is allergic to, according to several reports. Examples of these foods are cow's milk, other dairy products, eggs, fish, nuts, strawberries, and citrus fruit.

A recently published study describes a group of allergic mothers who avoided all cow's milk and instead used calcium tablets. These mothers obviously had far less cow's milk protein in their breast milk than did allergic mothers who drank cow's milk. A pediatrician who did not know which group the babies belonged to examined them and found that allergic eczema was much more rare among the babies not exposed to cow's milk protein during the last months in the womb or during the breastfeeding period.

Sandra decided to make an all-out effort. She stopped eating all foods to which she, her husband, or her first child was allergic, beginning roughly halfway through the pregnancy and continuing throughout the breastfeeding period. She watched like a hawk to make sure that her baby girl did not get even a drop of anything other than breast milk from the moment she was born. Sandra breastfed exclusively for six months and then introduced each new food in tiny portions. After this, she kept anything that she thought could cause an allergic reaction, including cow's milk, away from her baby until she was more than a year old. Sandra continued to also give breast milk at each meal. The last time I saw her, she proudly showed me a delightful little girl of almost two years with skin like a peach.

Sandra's son Matthew also looked great. He still had his allergies, but they had improved. In fact, Sandra maintained that smearing breast milk on his eczema helped. This is not inconceivable. Breast milk probably contains the gentlest fat available for lubrication and also suppresses inflammatory symptoms such as pain, irritation, swelling, and so on.

I cannot promise all families with allergies an equivalent story with a happy ending. Such a regime definitely helps some children, however. Depending on the seriousness of the problems your family has, you must decide how hard you want to try.

Asthma

Asthma, both with and without allergy, is less common among children who start life with only breast milk. Australian research following several thousand children from birth to school age recently showed a far lower risk of asthma among children who were exclusively breastfed, with all other milk kept away for at least the first four months. Unwarranted use of formula—sometimes even without the informed consent of parents—is still a problem in many maternity wards.

Diabetes in Babies and Young Children

When Carolyn was five years old, she was diagnosed with diabetes. Poor little girl, she had to stay in the hospital for a while. She was no longer allowed to eat what she wanted but instead had to keep to a diet. Every day was full of horrid shots to measure her blood sugar and to give insulin. The cells in her pancreas that should have made this hormone had been damaged in some way and didn't work anymore.

Carolyn's father, Harry, contacted me: "We are planning to have another baby," he said. "We have waited because there has been such a fuss with Carolyn. Now the people at the diabetes clinic say that Carolyn's diabetes may be connected with the fact that she was given cow's milk too early. Can this really be true?"

Harry felt uncomfortable because he had persuaded his wife to stop breastfeeding after a short time, with the best of intentions. He had thought breastfeeding was tiring for her and had wanted to contribute more to the feeding himself.

No one can answer this exactly with regard to Carolyn. There could be something to the theory, however. It has been proved that feeding cow's milk early in life to rats genetically susceptible to diabetes can provoke the disease. The advantages of exclusive initial breastfeeding come not only from the special properties in the breast milk; avoiding other food is also important.

Several reports now point to the too-early introduction of cow's milk to human infants as a risk factor for the development of diabetes in children. The sequence of events is suspected to be as follows: The newborn baby's intestinal wall is slightly "leaky" at the beginning, and large molecules therefore slip through. These include the molecules of cow's milk, which in some ways resemble molecules on the surface of the cells that should produce insulin.

Some babies given cow's milk protein eventually create antibodies against it. An antibody must suit what is being attacked, like a key to a lock. When the cow's milk antibodies meet an insulin-producing cell, it seems, they misunderstand it. They fasten to the cell because the surface is so like the surface of cow's milk protein. These cells are therefore destroyed. It is now believed that this is why babies given breast milk to start with have a lower risk of getting diabetes early in life. Studies from several countries show that this risk generally is reduced by 25 to 50 percent in breastfed babies.

The preventive effect of breast milk may be even greater when exclusive breastfeeding is achieved from the outset. Many babies believed to have been exclusively breastfed have in reality been given one or more bottles of cow's milk—based formula in the maternity or pediatric ward. In the 1980s, my research team and I found that 95 percent of all babies had been given one such bottle while there, often without the mother knowing about it. At that time, breastfeeding at night was not common. Staff cared for the babies in a nursery and did not want to leave them crying hour after hour without a feeding.

The length of the breastfeeding period also seems to have an effect. In both the United States and Finland, studies showed that the risk of developing diabetes decreased as the length of time for breastfeeding increased. Again, diabetes occurs for many reasons. Genetics play an important role. But even as a risk remains that your baby will develop diabetes, exclusive breastfeeding is one of the few things you can do yourself to reduce that risk.

I shared this knowledge with Carolyn's parents when they came for a consultation. I emphasized that even exclusive breastfeeding for the first six months and continued breastfeeding for the first two years could not guarantee to protect the new baby against diabetes. Heredity is a significant factor, and several family members had diabetes. It was worth the effort of breastfeeding to try to prevent it, however. The "preventive cure" is guaranteed to be harmless and is both healthy and enjoyable.

BOWEL DISEASE IN ADULTHOOD

If you were breastfed as a baby, it may benefit you into adulthood as well. Two serious bowel diseases that mainly affect younger adults, ulcerous colitis and Crohn's disease, lead to violent, frequent diarrhea—often with blood and mucus—due to a kind of inflammatory change of the intestines. The condition can become so serious that large parts of the bowel have to be removed.

Just as for diabetics, a research team found antibodies against cow's milk protein in the blood of patients with these bowel diseases. This finding has led to several studies on how these people were fed as babies. Again, as for diabetes, the diseases are less common in people who started life with breast milk than in those given cow's milk–based formulas as babies.

CANCER IN CHILDREN AND YOUNG PEOPLE

You might think that something with such a strong effect on the immune system as breast milk could also reduce the risk of cancer. A study from the state of Colorado looked into this. Researchers there compared 201 children with cancer to an equal number of healthy control group children with similar backgrounds in terms of age, gender, and dwelling place. The researchers found a slightly reduced risk among children who had been breastfed. This was especially clear with regard to cancer of the lymph glands, which occurred more frequently in children who had never been given breast milk. Much is still to be explained here, though. We do not really understand the possible effect mechanism, and we are waiting for confirmation.

Is This Only the Beginning?

New findings consistently indicate the long-term effects of breast milk. One research study of people with multiple sclerosis showed that fewer of them had been breastfed than had people in a comparable control group. If this holds true in future research, either the immune system or the fat layering of the central nervous system is probably involved.

Surgeons who transplant kidneys have also begun to realize the importance of breast milk. If you happen to be ill enough to require a kidney transplant, you will be lucky if your mother is the donor and if she used to breastfeed you. This appears to indicate that your immune system is slightly more like your mother's than like your father's, even though he is responsible for half of your genetic makeup. Your mother has probably transferred some permanent, extra immune factors to you through her breast milk. Because of this, the chance is greater that your body will accept her kidney more easily, rather than rejecting it as foreign.

You Have a Right to Know

This chapter has given you a few examples to illustrate a bit of what we know about the disease-preventing properties of breast milk. Remember, however, that even with a reduced risk, your baby can still fall ill. After all, people can drown with a lifejacket on.

Some parents may feel uncomfortable with the knowledge in this chapter. If you are a mother who has not breastfed your babies, you may be frightened. You may feel guilty or think that your baby will grow up to blame you for not providing breast milk. Even so, I think it is right to inform those without a medical background of these findings. After all, most reports appear as relatively complex scientific articles unintelligible to most people. Keeping important information secret from parents is to underestimate them. Only when you have enough knowledge can you make an informed choice—and giving your baby breast milk is something that most mothers can do with more or less effort.

If you are one of the few who cannot breastfeed, comfort yourself by reading chapter 16, and see how great things can still be!

Breast milk contains disease-preventing:

- Antibodies against bacteria and viruses.

- White blood cells—the body's police force.

- Lactoferrin, the protein that binds unhealthy, loose iron.

- Factors that promote the growth of benevolent bacteria in the bowel.

- Interferon, which fights viruses.

Breastfed babies are less likely to suffer from:

- Dangerous general infections in the neonatal period.

- Diarrhea and other diseases of the digestive system.

- Problems in the respiratory tract such as: common colds and infections with RS-virus, bronchitis, pneumonia, or ear infections.

- Urinary tract infections.

- Eczema and other allergies.

- Hypersensitivity to cow's milk proteins.

- Diabetes in childhood.

- Bowel disease in adulthood.

CHAPTER 13

. . .

Common Breastfeeding Problems

Many women experience discomfort or other problems during breastfeeding, especially to begin with. Fortunately, advice is available for ways to counter most of these problems.

ENGORGED BREASTS

When the milk kicks in seriously after a day or two, many women experience painful engorged breasts. This condition usually improves when the breasts have received adequate signals about how much milk the baby needs. The best way to get this across and to treat engorged breasts is to let the baby suck quite frequently but for a slightly shorter time. The baby then needs less at a time, and your breasts will not be stimulated to produce too much. By doing this, you will avoid problems with your breasts while supply and demand adjust to each other.

PLUGGED MILK DUCTS

When an area of the breast does not empty properly, it can feel tender and swollen. You may have a kink in one of your milk ducts, or pressure from your bra may have hindered free flow. Perhaps your baby did not suck vigorously enough to soften a hard, congested area full of milk.

This section must be emptied. First, make sure that the letdown reflex is elicited and the milk is getting out, preferably by allowing the baby to suck or by pumping the milk or expressing it manually. When the milk is flowing, massage the breast gently over the hard area in the direction of the nipple. You can use a little cream on your fingers so that you don't irritate the skin. Stroke firmly but gently,

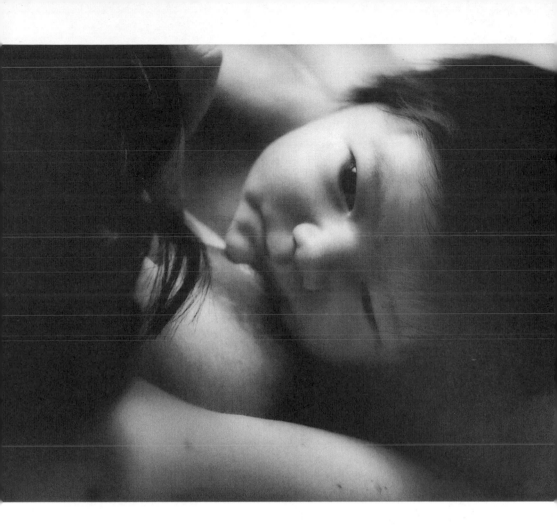

always toward the outlet. Do not stop until the area is soft. If you don't quite get there the first time, try again a little later.

MASTITIS

Infection of the breast, or mastitis, can occur if a swollen breast or plugged milk duct is left untreated and bacteria find their way there. The affected breast usually becomes hard, swollen, tender, hot, and red. You can run a high fever, perhaps even have an attack of the shivers. You feel dreadful!

Debra called me, completely desperate. She had been advised to empty her breast but couldn't get even a drop of milk out. Her husband had also tried to massage the breast, but the pain was unbearable. I advised Debra to take a hot bath. After a while, a little milk began to trickle out. She hung onto hope with this slight success and stayed in the tub for a long time, expressing the milk manually. She also felt that letting the breast float in the hot water really helped to relieve the pain. If you don't have a tub, try a hot shower, but because you are ill, be sure to sit comfortably. After the bath treatment, the painful breast was quite soft, and Debra's baby finished the job. Debra took a few paracetamol tablets and spent the next day sleeping, breastfeeding frequently, and expressing milk. By the end of two days, her problems had disappeared.

With early treatment, mastitis usually clears up after about twenty-four hours of expressing milk roughly every two hours during the day and a few times at night. If the baby cannot or will not suck enough, you must pump or express milk after having started the letdown reflex. The video *Breast Is Best* (see Resources, page 253) shows how to do this and how to take milk samples for cultivation of bacteria.

Things did not go as well for Heather. She had not managed to get any milk out and had not received any help. She also had a fever of over 102°F and went to the doctor. There she was given penicillin. Unfortunately, no milk sample was first taken. If a sample had been cultivated for a few days, it would have shown that Heather needed a completely different antibiotic. Angry staphylococci had attacked her, and her breast could not overcome these, probably because her milk was not being removed and the swelling breast tissue had eventually caused poor blood circulation. By the time I saw Heather, the mastitis had developed into a large abscess requiring surgery. She was admitted to the hospital, together with her baby. Heather was given a short-acting anesthetic, and we emptied more than 5 ounces of pus from her breast. Leaving the wound open, we inserted a rubber tube so that the abscess could continue to drain for as long as any pus remained. Alternatively, a catheter can be inserted into the abscess guided by ultrasound, without operating. The pus can then be suctioned out and the area flushed thoroughly. When repeated for several days, this procedure can produce good results with less discomfort for the mother than a surgical emptying.

Heather continued to breastfeed, even from the breast that had been operated on. No visible pus emptied through the nipple. To check this, drip some milk from both breasts onto a cotton ball and compare. The milk will soak into the cotton, while the pus will remain on the surface. The breastfeeding relieved the discomfort in her breast, in fact, and constant emptying promoted recovery. Milk leaked out through the wound for a short period, so Heather came back a few times. After her breast had healed, she continued to check it carefully. At the least sign of discomfort, she emptied it well and rested a lot. By doing this, she managed to hold in check several possible recurrences of breast inflammation.

Not everyone is so fortunate. Some women apparently have a tendency toward breast infections, usually following bad drainage and subsequent inflammation. Something in the breast may cause this. Often only one breast has problems—perhaps due to a narrow or crooked milk duct. I know several women who, because of repeated breast inflammation, have weaned off one breast and breastfeed only from the other. Breastfeeding with only one breast usually works well; after all, most women can produce enough milk for twins with two breasts. The weaning of one breast has to be done during a period without infection. When the milk is not emptied, the breast gradually stops producing. The process can be aided by applying gentle pressure on the breast after emptying.

Recurrent breast inflammation may be linked in some women to a slightly lowered level of immune response. I admire women who persevere and do not want to give up breastfeeding despite such problems. I sometimes give advice to stop: "You have battled on," I might say. "You have managed to give your baby a great start with breast milk for two months despite several severe cases of mastitis. Stop breastfeeding now."

I was waiting in line to see a movie in Oslo last year. Suddenly an unfamiliar woman came up to me and whispered triumphantly, "I didn't give up!" I looked really surprised until she explained that I had advised her to stop breastfeeding but that she had not wanted to. After many recurrences of mastitis, things had eventually worked out well for her. She and her baby had finally been rewarded with a marvelous, long, uncomplicated period of breastfeeding.

Thrush (or *Candida*)

For some women, breastfeeding is painful even if they do not have sore nipples. For some, the pain is not caused just by the first tender pulls on a full breast but rather continues after the baby has let go of the breast. This pain may be caused by a fungal infection of the breast. Thrush, *Candida albicans,* is especially common in pregnant women. The baby may become infected while moving through the birth canal if it gets the fungus in the mouth, then, infect the breast during suckling.

Once in a while, thrush is clearly visible in the mouth of the baby. At other times, there is no sign of fungus in either the mother or the baby, nor does it grow in a milk sample. Nonetheless, we often suspect fungus simply because of what the mother says. Yasmine's case was typical, as she described it: "It continues to hurt all the time while my baby is sucking and for a long time afterward. It feels as though someone is pulling a red hot steel wire in and out of my breast."

Some women are helped by simply smearing a thin layer of a non-prescription antifungal ointment or cream on the breast once it has been carefully air-dried after breastfeeding. Before the next feeding, some absorbent material is pressed against the breast to pick up any ointment residues. Do not rub, as this will tear the skin. If the pains persist or if the baby has thrush in the mouth, both mother and baby must be treated. See a doctor or seek advice from health services.

Cramp in the Nipple's Small Blood Vessels

The nipples of a few women suddenly change color from red to white accompanied by intense pain. This seems to be a kind of cramp in the nipple's tiny blood vessels and is usually triggered during stimulation of the nipple. Typically it follows a period of painful affliction of the breast, such as mastitis or *Candida*. Simple but effective advice for some mothers is to warm the breast well with a hot water bottle before feeding, for example. Strangely enough, others achieve a better effect by cooling the nipple. Otherwise, keeping the breast warm during the breastfeeding period is good general advice. Drinking a large cup of tea just before breastfeeding may also protect you from cramps. A lot of coffee, in contrast, can provoke cramping. Some women benefit from massaging and stimulating the breast for a good while before breastfeeding to carefully prepare the breast. Others find that the breast must be touched as little as possible apart from the baby's searching and sucking. Experiment to see what works for you.

Small doses of medicine to dilate the blood vessels can also alleviate cramping. A specialist must arrange this and follow up.

ECZEMA

Some women develop extreme eczema on their breasts, perhaps triggered by the often numerous ointments they have put on their breasts, in addition to the dampness from the milk. The skin becomes red with small bumps or blisters. If you have eczema, try applying a thin coat of the very mildest hydrocortisone cream after your breast has air-dried.

Naturally, the best thing to prevent moist skin is to walk around bare-breasted. When this is not practical, some women benefit from using a breast-cup inside their bra. Breast-cups with a perforated sheet at the top are the most comfortable against the skin. These collecting cups allow the nipple and areola to stand free in the air as they do when you are naked.

HOW DO I STOP USING A BREAST SHIELD?

Thin, soft breast shields can sometimes be useful, but as a rule, it is possible to solve a sucking problem without a shield. Breast shields are typically used for a couple of reasons: in spite of proper stimulation the nipple remains very flat and it is difficult for the baby to get hold of a large mouthful of breast, therefore the nipple of such a shield may make it easier for the baby to latch on. Also, very rarely the mother's nipples may be so sore that she can't stand for the baby to suck directly on her breast. But usually using a shield should be a last resort and is only a short-term solution. Because the breasts are not well stimulated through the shield, the baby may take in far less milk with the breast shield and often does not put on much weight. In addition, if you leave the hospital with a breast shield, you will often have major problems getting rid of it—so it is generally better not to use one in the first place.

Ask for help to stimulate a good rooting and latch-on. Always offer your baby the breast without a shield first. Try when your baby is sleepy or at least not already screaming with hunger. Use a few drops of milk on your nipple to tempt it. If your baby refuses to take the breast without a shield, try to cut a tiny piece off the tip of the shield every day. Allow your baby to search; don't force.

Breastfeeding After a Breast-Reduction Operation

Some women who have had breast-reduction surgery go on to have uncomplicated breastfeeding, but problems commonly follow such an operation. Surgeons try to preserve the ability to breastfeed, but this can be difficult. As a rule, plenty of glandular tissue is left to produce enough milk. Sometimes outlet ducts for the milk can be damaged or blocked by scar tissue, however. The operation can also affect the sensory nerves of the breast. When the baby sucks, messages are generally sent to the brain to indicate the need for oxytocin, which causes the letdown reflex. If this does not happen, the baby has major problems getting the milk out.

What you can do is to give breastfeeding a real chance. Follow all the good breastfeeding advice, starting out right after the birth if possible. Most women will then produce milk and feel that their breasts become full after two to four days. If your baby does not manage to get any milk out, you can ask for a hormone spray with synthetic oxytocin called Syntocinon. Sprayed up your nose before breastfeeding, Syntocinon has the same effect as oxytocin.

If this does not help, your outlet ducts are probably blocked. If you have really tried and not a single drop of milk has appeared after a few days, perhaps it is time to give up. Bind your breasts carefully (with a wide scarf, for example), pressing them gently against your body for a few days. They will gradually stop producing milk, and your body will slowly reabsorb what was already there. If this is uncomfortable, take a few painkillers. Tablets can also be given to stop your milk production—but these have side effects and do not always help unless given in the first twenty-four hours after delivery. You may be better off putting up with a few days of discomfort.

What if a little milk appears, but not enough? You must then consider whether to cope with double feeding, using both breasts and supplements. A little breast milk is obviously better than none. Some mothers who have undergone breast operations use an "artificial breast;" the baby suckles from the mother but at the same time gets formula through a thin plastic tube taped onto the breast. Chapter 16 tells more about this.

For some women, things gradually get better and better. Martina called me after she read in a newspaper that I was looking for people who had breastfed successfully after breast-reduction surgery. Martina's breasts had been operated on, and she told me that she had exclusively breastfed her third baby. For her first infant, she had had only a little milk but had managed to feed for six weeks. For her second, she had been even more motivated. Then she had breastfed for six months in addition to giving a bottle. "I was really encouraged to notice that the areas that were well-drained seemed to grow and gradually spread out, while the hard, full areas that were not emptied, eventually almost disappeared." After the birth of her third child, things went even better. "I breastfed him exclusively from when he was four weeks old. It was wonderful to feel like everyone else!"

Breastfeeding After a Breast Enlargement

A great deal has been written about silicone implants and their possible harmful effects. Recently there was a television program that led mothers with silicone implants to become terrified, and many called me. They were frightened because they had breastfed their babies.

It may be unhealthy for women to walk around with two large foreign objects made of silicone inside their bodies. With regard to breast milk, however, prevailing current opinion among experts worldwide is that it has not been proven that milk from a breast with an intact silicone implant contains silicone and whether, should it do so in some cases, this is harmful to health. It is certain, however, that both giving and being given breast milk has health benefits. Women with silicone implants are therefore advised to breastfeed.

Silicone is also found in pacifiers and in cow's milk (because of silicone in milking machines and tubes used in the dairy). Moisturizing creams and hair spray contain silicone. Because it does not irritate tissues, silicone is chosen in hospitals for catheters inserted into the body to remain there for a long time. Based on what is known today, most women with implants who are correctly informed will choose to breastfeed their babies.

Many plastic surgeons today use saline implants simply to avoid silicone. Breastfeeding problems are rarely encountered after insertion of an implant of any type. Some women with these implants must breastfeed more frequently at the outset, however, because they have slightly less room for storing milk. This is because they had small breasts to start with, and their skin may be extra taut after the implant. Nevertheless, the operation should not have disturbed the glandular tissue, and breastfeeding usually works well.

When the Baby Rejects the Breast

Many babies gradually wean themselves from the breast at around one year of age. They eat a lot of other food; the mother's milk comes slowly, in smaller quantities; they are bored as they lie facing their mother when the world outside is so exciting. The baby does not need breast milk any longer, and this is great.

Worse is when a small baby suddenly does not want to take the breast anymore and goes on strike. This may happen because of a sickness, such as an earache or a blocked nose, or because the baby has experienced pain or has been frightened while in the suckling position, or because the mother smells unfamiliar due to perfume, soap, smoke, alcohol, menstruation, and so on. In this case, you must be patient. Try to offer the breast when the baby is sleepy or when everything is peaceful. Hold your baby in a new position—for example, allow the baby to "stand" while sucking. Search for the cause. Try to carry your baby around, your breast naked and a drop of milk next to your little one's mouth. Do not force your baby; allow your baby to try again in time. A sucking strike can be frustrating but almost always passes after a while. In the meantime, express a little milk and give it to your baby in a cup.

Being Away from Your Breastfed Baby: Expressing and Storing Milk

Suppose you must start to work again or will be gone on a trip—but you want your baby to be given breast milk while you are away. Many mothers simply collect drip-milk over time. Use a bowl-shaped breast-cup inside your bra on one breast while feeding from the other. These cups are available at drugstores or from your healthcare provider. Milk usually drips while your baby is sucking. If not, you can express a little milk when your baby is well under way at one breast. Right after you have finished feeding, empty the milk into a small container and put it in the freezer. If the volume is small, pour the fresh milk on top of the frozen until you have enough for a feeding. If you need a bigger quantity, pump or express milk manually.

Fresh breast milk can be kept in the refrigerator for two days. Milk thawed after freezing can be kept for one day. Breast milk can be frozen for three months. After this, its flavor can change and it loses some of its valuable properties—but it is not harmful. The main problem is that it might go rancid. Smell and taste the milk yourself to see if this has happened.

Thaw the milk slowly. Take care when using a microwave, which may cause uneven heating. Always shake thoroughly before use, and be aware that some of the milk's disease-fighting properties will be lost when a microwave is used.

BITING

Some babies will try biting the nipple while breastfeeding. This is very painful and most mothers react spontaneously by exclaiming and pulling the baby off the breast. Usually that's enough to show the little one that biting simply is not acceptable. If not, try pulling the baby very close the next time biting occurs. A wide-open full mouth makes it virtually impossible to bite.

PREGNANT AGAIN: DO I HAVE TO STOP BREASTFEEDING?

You can continue to breastfeed even if you become pregnant again. Sometimes the baby will reject the breast, perhaps due to a change in the taste of the milk, and some women have very tender breasts at the beginning of their pregnancy. If both mother and baby want to continue, though, that's fine—as long as the mother gets enough nourishment for herself, the growing fetus, and her milk production, and as long as she does not feel too tired.

Some women react with premature contractions to the breast stimulation of feeding. This tendency increases as you get further into the pregnancy, and you may need to stop breastfeeding to avoid a premature birth. Also, if you are not sure that you want to breastfeed both babies simultaneously, stopping in good time before the birth is sensible.

Tandem Breastfeeding

If you choose to continue breastfeeding throughout your pregnancy, the milk changes and colostrum still forms when you give birth. Remember that the newborn baby must be given priority. Some small older brothers and sisters take great joy in being given the leftovers. In some families, each baby has one breast after a while. This can be one way for a mother to handle an otherwise jealous, unruly eighteen-month old when alone with her babies.

If you suspect that you will feel disgust at letting your older child feed at your breast after the new baby has finally arrived, it is probably kindest to wean the first child in good time beforehand. Mammals in general do not usually breastfeed several litters at the same time.

Some common breastfeeding problems that can usually be solved are:

- Overfull—engorged—breasts.

- Plugged milk ducts.

- Mastitis—an inflammation or infection of the breast.

- Pains in the breast caused by fungus.

- Cramps in the small blood vessels in the nipple.

- Eczema and sore skin on the breast.

- Breastfeeding after breast operations.

- A baby who will not suckle.

- Being away from your baby for a few hours.

CHAPTER 14

. . .

The Pacifier: Friend or Foe?

Guy was an energetic, breastfed baby. He sucked with concentration and took plenty of milk. Nonetheless, he was often a little fretful. He wanted to suck at the breast most of the time. In the end, his mother couldn't stand it. After three weeks, she gave him a pacifier. Peace descended over the home.

Breastfeeding continued without problems. Guy continued to put on weight, just as he ought to do, until he was around six weeks old. Then, suddenly, he stopped gaining weight. Even though he was happy when he had something to suck on, he fretted and cried more. His parents ran to and fro with his pacifier. What had happened?

Because Guy was getting bigger, he needed more food. And how should he get his mother's breasts to produce more milk? By sucking more than usual. How could he get more time at the breast? By crying!

Guy was trying his best. He cried and fretted when his body signaled that he needed more food. But his mother's breasts weren't getting the message. Instead, his parents translated his signals incorrectly and gave him a pacifier. Milk production stayed at the same level, and Guy's weight also remained static.

GIVING THE BREAST THE MESSAGE

The only advice I gave Guy's parents was to put the pacifier away for two weeks and to put him to the breast whenever he wanted it. After a few weeks, I saw them again. The mother's breasts were full. Guy's weight had begun to normalize. He was calmer. The parents went home happy. They hadn't decided to throw out the pacifier. They wanted to keep it in reserve. But they now were aware that

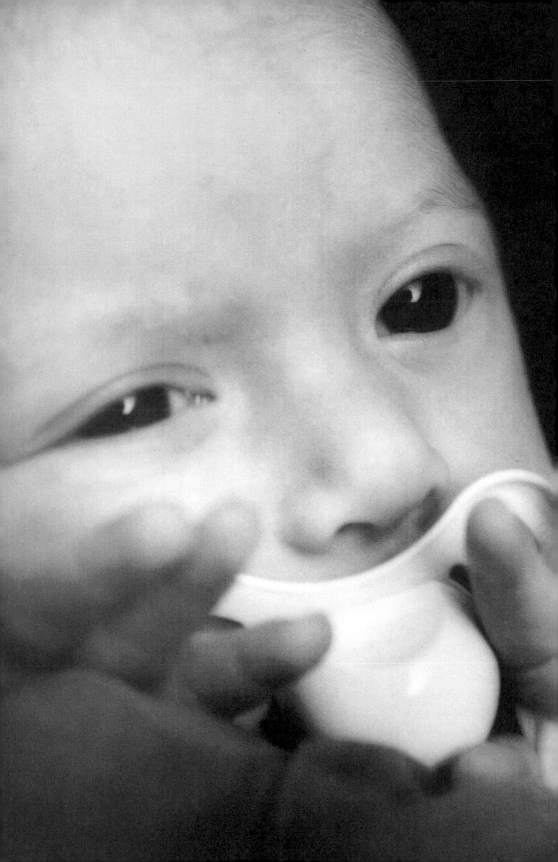

every once in a while some days of extra breastfeeding would be required as their baby boy grew.

This is one reason for using a pacifier with caution. The longer the total breastfeeding time per day, the higher the levels of the hormone prolactin. (This Latin word translates "for the milk.") Prolactin is important for regulating the amount of milk, especially at the start of breastfeeding. Sucking on a pacifier takes stimulation time away from the breast.

Emptying the breast properly is another way to signal the need for increasing production. The more milk that is removed, the more will be made for the next time. An energetic baby who sucks vigorously and drinks all the milk stored in the breast gives a strong signal to increase production. If a baby sucks weakly and leaves behind a half-full breast, the breast will reduce production, even if the baby actually needs more food. Many women who have had more than one child say that their breasts feel different according to the intensity of the new baby's sucking. Babies who suck weakly—premature babies, for example—can be stimulated to make a more productive effort. See chapter 7 for more information.

Nipple Confusion

One mother wrote me an indignant letter. Here is a small excerpt: "Our little girl was a fine healthy baby when she was born, but rather small. She clung to my breasts like a leech and seemed content to be there. After a few days, the maternity nurse found out that the baby's weight had gone down, and she was given a bottle of milk supplement. When I tried to feed the baby afterward, she had changed. She would not take the breast, even though I had plenty of milk. At first, I thought it was because she was full, but even later she wouldn't take the breast in the same way as she did just after she was born. It seemed like she couldn't open her mouth properly. She just lay with her mouth almost closed and tugged on my nipple until I bled. I was about to give up breastfeeding completely. Thanks to my experienced sister, I held out, but it took weeks before the baby started sucking well again. Afterward I learned that you shouldn't give a pacifier or a bottle to a newborn baby, as this can complicate breastfeeding. Do you think that one bottle of milk could be the reason for these problems? I'm really furious with the hospital."

Maybe this little girl suffered from what we call "nipple confusion." Previously, supplements in the maternity ward were normally given by spoon. It was well known that a breastfed baby was not to be given a bottle because doing so might lead to sucking problems. When I travel around the world and lecture at hospitals, I ask the older staff when this advice fell out of fashion and when bottles started being given instead. This appears to have happened sometime in the 1970s.

More recent research proves this old wisdom to be true: a newborn baby who sucks on a long, rigid nipple—whether a pacifier or a bottle nipple—may have problems taking the breast properly. There may be several reasons for this. One is that the position of the baby's jaw is quite different when sucking from the breast than when sucking from a bottle.

Hamburgers or Spaghetti?

Carry out a little experiment on yourself: put your thumb into your mouth and tickle the roof of your mouth. This action stimulates the sucking reflex. Note how you keep your mouth almost shut, or pursed, when you suck your thumb. This is more or less what happens when a baby sucks on a pacifier or bottle.

Now try to suck on the softest part of your underarm, so hard that you can feel it right up in the roof of your mouth. You won't be able to manage this because your arm is not a breast with a nipple. But note how your mouth gapes really widely as you try to do this. This is the shape of the newborn baby's mouth who is breastfeeding well.

The shape of the mouth when sucking on an artificial nipple may be compared to the mouth's shape when sucking on spaghetti. At the breast, however, the shape of the mouth should be the same as if you were trying to eat an enormous hamburger.

Many newborn babies manage the technique of sucking both on a pacifier and from the breast. Some get very confused, however. The problem is that we cannot know in advance which baby will have problems with breastfeeding after having been given a pacifier or a bottle. Even a single bottle of milk given in a maternity ward has been shown to slightly increase the risk that breastfeeding problems will occur.

Babies fed intravenously or by tube, with the milk going right into the stomach, may benefit from a pacifier. Sucking helps the digestion. Besides, babies love to suck, and these babies have no other opportunity to do so. In this case, it is necessary to weigh the advantages against the risk of having problems with sucking when the baby is finally put to the breast. If you think your baby will be able to suck from your breast in just a few days, maybe you should keep the pacifier away.

Wait Before Using Superstimuli

The general rule is that a baby should learn to suck at the breast before being given any type of pacifier or artificial nipple. Breastfeeding should be well established, and the mother should have plenty of milk. In practice, this is normally around two weeks after birth.

If a breastfed baby must be given food in another way, use a little spoon or cup or a syringe without a needle. Sit the baby almost upright on your lap, and pour a little milk at a time on the upper side of the lower lip, not down the throat. Some babies will simply drink it, while others will lap up the milk like a kitten, using the lips and tongue. Thus, nipple-sucking confusion is avoided. Wrapping the baby in a baby blanket—swaddling—in advance might be sensible. Less milk will be spilled.

The strong, constant stimulation of the roof of the mouth from a firm, artificial nipple functions as a kind of superstimulus, making the baby almost insensitive to the soft, natural stimulus from the breast. This is similar to the way in which a dog—or a child—who is used to strict, shouted orders will not react to quiet, gentle requests.

Ultrasound pictures sometimes show a fetus sucking energetically on its thumb. The same is observed among newborn babies who put their fingers in their mouths with a dexterity that indicates plenty of practice. I have noted many times that these finger-sucking infants more often seem to have problems sucking strongly on the breast. Perhaps they are giving themselves the superstimulus that interferes with sucking from the breasts.

Bottle Feeding Is Harder Work

It was once believed that babies used less energy to suck from a bottle than to suck from the breast. Modern research shows, however, that the opposite is true. Breastfeeding is less demanding, even for weak, premature babies. Because of the letdown reflex, milk drips and sometimes runs into a baby's mouth after a while of sucking. If the stream of milk becomes too much, the baby can reduce it by pressing around the soft areola or by pushing the tongue against the nipple where the milk is pouring out. In this way, the baby can take a breather while feeding without losing grip on the breast.

When drinking from a bottle, the baby normally has to suck actively the whole time in order to get the milk. If the nipple has a too large hole, on the other hand, the milk flows quickly and almost by itself. It can then be difficult for the baby to stop the stream of milk because the flow is faster than from the breasts and because the bottle nipple cannot be compressed so easily. It is thus more difficult for the baby to breathe while sucking from the bottle. Altogether, the technique is rather different. Right at the start, when the baby should be practicing on a soft almost empty breast, using a bottle might be particularly confusing. The bottle delivers milk immediately, and the baby gets the impression that this type of sucking leads to results.

Position of the Teeth

A while ago I took part in a television debate about pacifiers. A camera crew had filmed children at a day care center, and nearly all the babies had pacifiers. An expert from the Dental College told of new research that indicates that babies who use pacifiers run an increased risk of later having crooked teeth and thus requiring braces. I was asked whether modern, busy parents these days replace love and care with pacifiers. Pure rubbish, of course. Modern parents are no less fond of their children than parents in earlier generations. They simply know of this contraption that can frequently offer a bit of peace and quiet. I must admit that my own children used pacifiers, and two of them needed braces.

Limiting Pacifier Use

Maybe we should use common sense and at least try to limit the use of the pacifier. First, see whether the baby calms down with feeding, rocking, singing, massage, a dry diaper, or being carried. All these experiences in addition stimulate the baby. The pacifier only makes the baby passive. Of course, this is sometimes marvelous.

If you do use a pacifier, boil it now and then. This is not because the baby will suffer from bacteria. Sometimes, however, the baby develops thrush, or fungal infection, in the mouth and can pass it on to the breast, causing pain for the mother. The pacifier can act as a source of new infection even after both mother and baby have been treated.

An older baby will be able to stick the pacifier in its mouth without help. That is, if it knows where to find the pacifier. Tie the pacifier to the baby's bed so it can be found easily; this will save you from waking up a few times at night. The baby will learn to connect the pacifier with bed and sleep, and you will not end up with a large child tottering around with a pacifier at all times of day and night. Make sure that the ribbon is short enough that it cannot possibly get caught around the baby's neck; it should be a maximum of 4 inches. Treat the baby to one pacifier for each side of the bed. With a very short ribbon, also, the pacifier will fall out of the mouth once the baby has fallen asleep and turned over a bit. Thus the baby will not get used to having a pacifier in the mouth continuously while asleep. This will reduce the risk of affecting the amount of time with pressure on the teeth as well. My youngest child loved her bedtime pacifier with its short silk ribbon and a lock of Mommy's hair and sometimes got into bed in the daytime just to be cozy or to comfort herself when life wasn't going her way.

Avoid bottles and pacifiers completely until:

- The baby has learned to suck well at the breast.

- The amount of milk is stable and sufficient.

The use of pacifiers can:

- Lead to nipple confusion and breastfeeding problems.

- Prevent signals for increased milk production as the child grows.

- Pacify the child, who may then miss natural stimuli.

- Lead to repeated fungal infections.

- Lead to crooked teeth.

- Make the baby wake up every time the pacifier falls from the mouth.

CHAPTER 15

. . .

When Is it Necessary to Supplement Mother's Milk?

The answer is short and sweet: supplementation is seldom necessary in the first six months. As usual, however, the human being's large brain and meddlesome behavior have led us off track for many years. For several decades up to around 1975 formula was given routinely to all babies in Norwegian maternity wards. Eventually doubt increased that giving human babies milk from a completely different species of mammal during the first few months of life might not be ideal. After that, sugar water was given instead.

In the beginning of the 1980s, I was steadily becoming better positioned to do something about breastfeeding in hospitals. As a resident in the obstetrics/gynecology department in one of Norway's largest maternity wards, I did the rounds with new mothers there.

"How is the breastfeeding going?" I would ask them.

"Not very well," they would answer, often in tearful voices.

"Not going well?" I asked in dismay. "Why not?" At that time, the old routine was finally beginning to relax. Mothers were allowed to breastfeed more often and even to give both breasts if they wanted to.

"The baby won't suck from my breast," whispered the mothers, their heads bowed.

"Why won't the babies take the breast?" I asked the midwives and the maternity nurses.

"Oh, they are probably feeling a bit nauseated," would be the answer, with all the weight of experience. This may sound rather strange, but anyone who has seen a newborn baby push away the breast, gulp up the milk, and look sick would know immediately what they meant.

No More Sugar Water

This set off my first research project, a study of 400 mothers and their newborn infants. The results showed that a healthy, full-term baby would be given on average 20 ounces of sugar water during the first three days of life. This might not sound so terrible, but if you calculate the relative amount an adult man would drink in relation to his body weight, you will find this equivalent to more than 40 bottles of soft drinks!

In spite of this, hospital staff were wondering why babies were so uninterested in the breast. There were several reasons: The babies had been sucking regularly on a bottle, so their need to suck was not particularly acute. They had been given masses of liquid and were not thirsty. They were getting plenty of calories and were not hungry. In addition, the sugar water was mixed according to taste and often was so sweet that it would have made anyone feel sick.

With a team, I carried out the study and wrote two scientific papers about this. The first called "One Week on Milk and Water" was published in the journal of the Norwegian Medical Association. An article in English was later published on the follow-up of the two test groups: those who had been given sugar water and those who had been given only breast milk. According to the follow-up, the group given sugar water was breastfed for a shorter period in total than the group given only milk from the mother's breast.

I like to think that this study helped to ensure that today healthy, full-term, newborn babies are rarely given anything other than their mother's milk. When we actually stopped the routine use of formula, sugar water, and even boiled water, no more babies than before had a low blood sugar level or became jaundiced or dehydrated. It was also shown that the babies given breast milk alone actually weighed a little more after five days than did those given sugar water as well. This was because the mothers of babies not given sugar water were now breastfeeding earlier and more often, thus producing breast milk more quickly and in greater quantities than the mothers of babies given sugar water.

Most Babies Are Equipped to Wait for Their Mother's Milk

A well-nourished baby born at the end of a full-term pregnancy has a built-in supply of food. The baby lives off a large supply of sugar in the liver until the mother's milk really comes in. In addition, full-term babies usually have a solid layer of fat under their skin. This is why they are so nice and chubby.

A story is told of a baby found many days after an earthquake by the side of his dead mother among the ruins. Everything indicated that the baby had been born immediately after the disaster. He had not received any food since he was born. Nonetheless, he was in relatively good physical shape, because he had drawn on the sugar reserves in his liver and on the fat under his skin. This is an extreme case, of course, but most newborn babies will manage perfectly well without nourishment for a few days.

Furthermore, most mothers start to produce milk earlier than they did a few decades ago. This is because the baby is put to the breast to suck right after birth and later as often as it indicates an interest, which is usually very often in the beginning.

We try never to forget the breastfeeding "disaster" that occurred a generation ago as a result of the unnatural routines practiced then. At that time, mothers were separated from their babies right after birth. The baby was not put to the breast on the first day. One reason given was that the milk might go down the wrong way. Another was that there wasn't any mother's milk yet anyway.

Subsequently, mothers were allowed to feed their babies only for twenty minutes every four hours. The baby was allowed to feed only from one breast at a time, and not during the night. If you yourself didn't receive breast milk when you were a baby, it may be because of these routines. Chances are that your mother would have liked to breastfeed. Instead of upbraiding her, ask her to read this and tell her it wasn't her fault. On the whole, only those endowed by nature to become particularly big producers managed to breastfeed successfully at that time.

Most maternity wards now consider giving a supplement only when a baby has lost around 10 percent of its birth weight. But by then someone should have noticed the tendency and done something about it. If the baby does not stop losing weight in a reasonable amount of time, a knowledgeable person should observe the breastfeeding routine. Are the mother and baby comfortable so that breastfeeding is not cut short because of discomfort? Does the baby have its mouth latched well onto the breast? If these things look all right, the mother and baby may need an extra day or two in the maternity ward, with necessary help and increased rest. This normally solves the problem.

A baby given a supplement that's not really needed, however, may lose the motivation to suck, which is necessary to stimulate the breasts to produce milk. Well-meaning people who give an unnecessary bottle in the maternity ward may thus be doing both mother and baby an unintentional disservice. The intention is to help the poor little baby, who is screaming so much and looks so hungry, or to relieve the mother so she can sleep without having to wake up to feed. The results can be long-term problems or breastfeeding failure from the start.

Most women who have given birth for the first time begin to produce milk in earnest about three days after the birth. For mothers of a subsequent child, the milk often comes in earlier. But life is not fair. For some people, the process takes longer, often because of a difficult beginning. From time to time, I even meet women such as this fourth-time mother, who said, "I don't have enough milk until a week's gone by. Now that I know this, I can relax. The first time, there was a lot of fuss in the maternity ward, and it made me panic. This time we give the baby just what he needs as a supplement, but I let him suckle a lot from me, too." She was quite right; after six days, her breasts were starting to produce plenty of milk.

As part of the work to make Norwegian delivery rooms and maternity wards more baby-friendly, guidelines indicate which of the full-term babies healthy enough to stay with their mothers in the maternity ward will need supplements. Many of the country's leading neonatologists from university hospitals were involved in drawing up these guidelines.

The main rule is that a supplement should be given only on medical advice—that is, when the doctor has ordered it. Such medical advice might be given for small babies who have not grown as they should in the womb, or for very large babies who are slightly more susceptible to lower blood sugar, which can, in the worst case, lead to seizures and other problems. These babies cannot always manage to wait until the breast milk comes in. They should also be put to the breast and have their mothers' milk when available, however, because breast milk is best. Occasionally, a supplement is given for "pacifying reasons." That is, an inconsolable baby with a worn-out mother may be given a supplement just once, without a bottle. This is seldom necessary when the baby is with the mother and can suck from her at regular intervals, however.

SUPPLEMENTS AFTER YOU GET HOME

If you go home with a baby who hasn't started to put on weight since birth, do not wait too long to get the baby weighed, either at the well-baby clinic, your doctor's office, or at the hospital. Sometimes a baby has to get over a hurdle of disquiet and minimal weight increase before breastfeeding starts to work, and this must be monitored carefully.

Eventually the baby will start to put on weight, even if he or she is not exactly following the weight charts for average growth the whole time. If the baby still isn't putting on weight after the first few days, you must get help to check the cause. Is the problem in the breast-feeding technique or in too brief or infrequent feedings? Is the baby jaundiced, listless, or sick? Whatever the cause, you will both probably benefit from some extra days with plenty of rest, food and drink for you, and with more frequent and prolonged breastfeeding. Sometimes other solutions are necessary.

Paul's mother's breasts were full of milk every morning, while there was very little milk in the evening. Then he sucked even more lustily and for longer, so her breasts were stimulated to even greater production the next morning. She could not manage to reverse this up and down trend and also needed time to look after her other children in the evening. She sorted it out like this: In the morning, when there was plenty of time and she had a lot of milk, she hand-milked a good quantity of the extra rich hindmilk, the "after" milk. She put this in the refrigerator until evening. Then the father would top Paul up with these precious drops of milk by cup feeding after normal breastfeeding, while the mother read to the other children. Sometimes they followed this option during the night as well if the mother was really tired.

Sandra, another mother, had a good start to breastfeeding, but after three months, her baby suddenly stopped putting on weight. He had begun to sleep through the night during the previous few weeks. Sandra thought this was wonderful, of course, but decided she would rather return to breastfeeding at night again than start up with bottles and formula. This was sensible. The amount of milk increased considerably, the baby put on weight, and the problem was solved. No big surprise: The breastfeeding hormone prolactin is actually at its top level when the baby feeds at night; this benefits milk production for the next day. Of course, feeding during the night is not necessary if your baby sleeps through the night and is also putting on weight, as long as you do not have a tendency to plugged milk ducts or mastitis and you are not using exclusive breastfeeding as a form of contraception during the first six months. You can read about this in chapter 20.

If sufficient and proper help is given and good advice followed, most mothers can produce enough milk for their baby. For a few women, however, this is impossible, including women who are seriously ill and need to take strong medication and some of those who have had operations on their breasts, to make them smaller, for example.

When a supplement must be given, the way in which it is done is important. If only a small volume is to be given, a small cup or spoon is best used. The method is described at the end of this chapter. So as not to cause nipple confusion in the baby, avoid bottles.

Be aware that the amount of breast milk you produce will normally go down if you start giving supplements regularly. This is because the baby will no longer suck quite as much on the breasts.

Giving mixed feedings is exhausting. Sometimes this is the only solution, however. People who manage to give both breast milk and supplements often make a huge investment.

If you need to give your baby anything other than breast milk on a permanent basis, or if you're not going to breastfeed at all, it is best to use bottles.

When Can the Baby Eat Solids?

Grace normally has very small breasts and was delighted with her new figure when she was breastfeeding. She had to feed her baby often, however, sometimes every hour during the daytime. Perhaps the room for storage was limited. Eventually she felt that life was just one long feeding. As far as I could see, she was doing everything that could be done, and her baby was sucking energetically. He was quite long for his age, but slim. When he was four months old, Grace began to give him small amounts of solids.

Babies should not have anything except milk until they are four months old—and it is probably best to breastfeed completely for the first six months. Clearly women differ, however. Some are naturally big producers. Others really have to struggle to produce enough milk. Grace continued to breastfeed before giving her baby other food, feeding her baby exclusively breast milk.

The ideal time to start giving solids seems to be around six months. By this time, babies are sufficiently developed to be able to "chew," swallow, and digest food. They start trying to grab food and stick it into their mouths. If babies are not given the chance at this age, getting them to eat solids may be difficult later on. Just as for potty training, there appears to be a special time when babies are ready to eat "real" foods. Then the baby must be given the opportunity. Around this time, many babies also need the extra iron found in various solids. Up until the age of six months, breastfeeding is the best way to protect most babies against anemia. This is because the iron in the mother's milk is so easily digestible and easily absorbed by the baby's gut. If the mothers choose only to breastfeed past the first six months, however, some babies will have a low blood count.

Many babies still exclusively breastfed after six months, without other types of food, put on less weight than children with a more varied diet. There is thus no special advantage to exclusive breastfeeding for more than six months. On the other hand, it is important that the baby continues to receive breast milk in combination with other food throughout the entire first year of life.

Indications are that it might be advantageous to introduce all forms of new food slowly, in tiny tastes, under the cover of plenty of breast milk. This practice mimics that of other mammals. Today this careful introduction of solids is considered to contribute to protection against both allergies and celiac disease, a gluten intolerance. In Sweden, babies are commonly given liquid gruel at an early stage, and speculation is that this measure has led to an increase in celiac disease.

ORDINARY COW'S MILK?

Some people don't want their baby to have cow's milk before it is necessary and therefore use their own breast milk for making baby

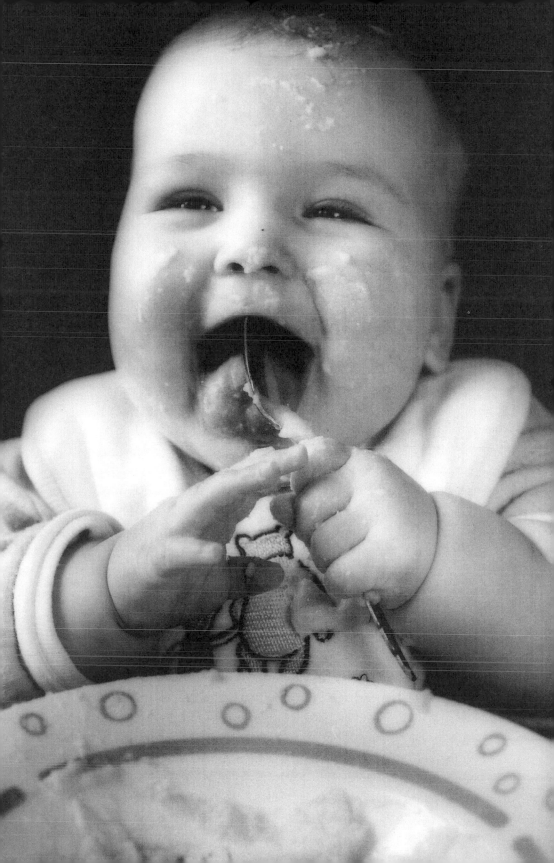

porridge. This is perfectly fine, of course, and helps the transition to other foods. If you don't have excess milk or can't face doing this, however, you can mix the porridge with water or formula. Pediatricians and nutritionists are currently discussing when a baby can start to have cow's milk like the rest of the family. A study a few years ago showed that some of the children in a group given cow's milk before they were one year old had minute intestinal bleeding, which was not found among a control group of children given formula, even though formula is produced from cow's milk.

Following this, some doctors recommended waiting until a baby is a year old before giving cow's milk. Not everybody agrees with this, however. If you choose to give cow's milk during your baby's second six months, it's a good idea to heat it to a boil. This splits some of the biggest proteins and makes the milk more easily digestible.

Before you give a supplement in the first four to six months:

- Check that you have followed all the advice in order to continue exclusive breastfeeding.

- Consider the additional work of using bottles, compared to taking more time to breastfeed.

Some tips for giving liquid supplements are:

- Let the baby sit almost upright.

- Try wrapping the baby's arms in a baby blanket.

- Use a little cup, a soft plastic medicine cup, or a spoon.

- Put the edge of the cup or spoon right against the baby's lower lip.

- Let the liquid come into contact with the baby's tongue.

- Ideally, let the baby lap up the milk with the tongue and lip movements.

- Don't pour in so much at one time that it goes down the wrong way.

When the baby is ready for solids:

- Start with little tastes.

- Introduce one type of food at a time; wait a bit before introducing the next food.

- Give breast milk at every mealtime, ideally before any other food.

CHAPTER 16

. . .

Bottle Babies

There are a number of possible reasons for not breastfeeding. Perhaps you started to breastfeed, but complications or circumstances in your life made it necessary for you to stop. Maybe because of an illness you have to take strong medicines that get into your milk. Maybe you have had a breast-reduction operation and can't produce milk as a result. Maybe you have adopted your newborn baby.

Currently, ninety-nine out of every one hundred mothers in Norway breastfeed their babies following birth. After three months, around ninety percent are still breastfeeding. Because breastfeeding has become so common, it feels all the worse not to breastfeed your baby. Some women feel they are considered second-class mothers and notice negative reactions from others when they take out a bottle instead of a breast.

This is incredibly sad. I was asked on television about the problem of the pressure to breastfeed and used the opportunity to say, straight into the camera, "If you see a mother give a bottle to a tiny baby, please be aware that she probably has a very good reason for not breastfeeding her baby. Don't make it difficult for her with remarks or looks. She is just as good a mother as all the others!"

Very few women in Norway voluntarily make the choice not to breastfeed. Those who do make this decision can be women with a network of friends and relatives who convince them that breastfeeding is just trouble. If you are one of these, take a look at the chapters on breastfeeding and breast milk before you make a final decision. Occasionally, the choice not to breastfeed is based on mental health problems. I have encountered a victim of incest who could not tolerate having her breasts touched in any situation. Whatever your reason, if

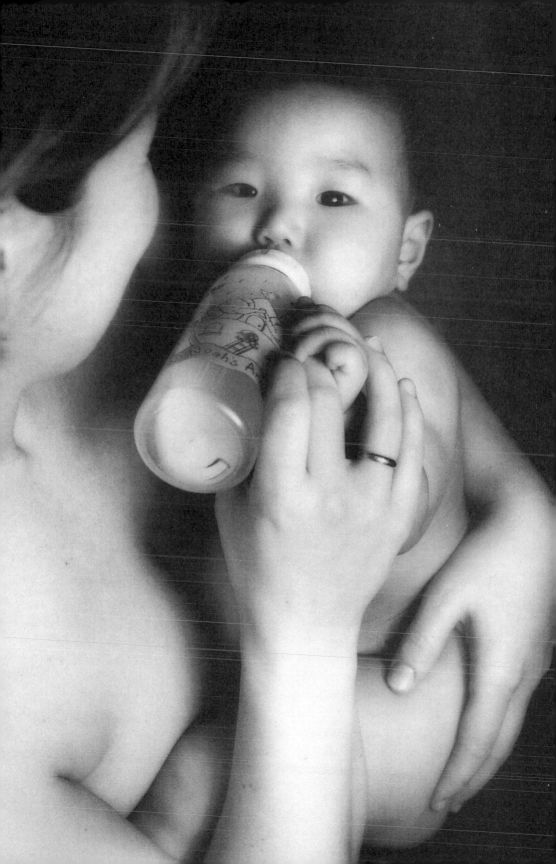

your baby is going to be fed with a bottle, totally or partially, try to include the elements that come naturally during breastfeeding.

INTERPLAY AND CLOSENESS WHEN FEEDING

Tilly and Ben got in touch with me before they traveled to Colombia to collect their adopted baby boy. They had heard that even adoptive mothers could breastfeed. This is true, particularly if the breasts have developed in an earlier pregnancy and if the baby still is intensely eager to suck. This was not the case for Tilly. Her little Karl Juan was going to be a bottle-fed baby.

Tilly and Ben had longed for this baby. They had thought a lot about the feedings and planned to imitate the breastfeeding situation as much as possible. Tilly held the baby close to her own body, and Ben did the same when it was his turn. Karl Juan would feel the warmth and the breathing movements from a big body while he fed. They held him in such a way that he could see a loving adult face the whole time. They chatted to him. His cheek always lay against naked skin: a bare arm or a chest where he could feel a heart beating. After a while, Karl Juan began to stroke his parents' skin with his small hands. He enjoyed the safe smell of a human body from familiar armpits.

Instead of a pacifier, Tilly and Ben let Karl Juan suck on a clean adult finger when he was unsettled, wanting him to have contact with human skin also in his mouth. Tilly even put him to her breast. He wasn't particularly interested, having had no experience of that sort of thing. She smeared a little milk on her nipple. Later she tried with something sweet. Eventually he would suck for a while, looking at her in amazement. "The most difficult thing about letting him use my breasts for comfort sucking was that everyone else thought I was crazy," wrote Tilly, in a long letter telling me how things have gone. "They thought I had wanted a baby for such a long time that I had gone completely mad and that I was trying to convince myself that I was going to breastfeed. But I only told them that the mouth is a sensitive area, which could also benefit from skin-to-skin contact. Furthermore, it might even be good for his teething. But I ended up only offering him my breast for comfort when we are at home alone."

Several adoptive mothers I know use a nursing supplement, or "Lact aid." This is a flat plastic bottle that hangs around the neck. A thin tube runs out of this and is fastened to the breast. The sucking baby gets both the formula from the nursing supplement and whatever milk has formed in the actual breast. The tube can also be put into a bottle or a cup. One such mother who had breastfed a few years earlier found after a few weeks that she had enough milk to exclusively breastfeed her adopted child for a while. Most use ordinary bottles with nipples, however, and are quite happy with this.

There are indications that bottle-fed babies do not develop quite as well in every respect as breastfed babies. Whatever small differences exist may partly be due to the fact that that some bottle-fed babies lack the stimuli that breastfed babies get automatically. Old studies agree with this—for example, studies from institutions where babies are left with a bottle, propped up against a pillow, alone in their beds. Even some worn-out parents today might be tempted to do this when things are difficult. But for the most part, such practices should be avoided. The baby needs warmth and stimulation, skin and eye contact, good sounds, and the smell of a human body at every single meal.

Eighteen-year-old "Samantha" couldn't manage this. She had a lot to cope with herself. She had been dependent on drugs when she became pregnant but had managed to come off them and was allowed to keep her baby. The baby was irritable and demanding after the birth. Samantha thought breastfeeding was messy and tiring and quickly gave up. After she went home, the mother and baby were followed up with care. The baby was developing poorly, and we wondered if he had a brain injury. Then it appeared that Samantha was lethargic and disinterested when she fed her baby. She didn't talk to him or cuddle him. She often left him in his stroller with a bottle so that she could have a little peace. When she was given help, however, and taught how to feed the baby while making contact and stimulating him, the baby began to show that he enjoyed it. Samantha became happier herself and more interested in her little one after she had been taught to understand his response. Things are now going quite well for them both, even though they still need support.

FORMULA

Babies do grow up fine without a drop of mother's milk. As one big, sturdy young man from the north of Norway, who didn't agree that breastfeeding was so important, said, "Just look at me. I didn't have a nipple in my mouth until I was engaged to be married!"

Modern breast milk substitutes, known as formulas, are based on cow's milk, specially treated and adapted to be easily digestible and beneficial for human babies. Iron, minerals, and vitamins are added. The large milk proteins are broken down into smaller proteins. Up until 1996, Norwegian breast milk substitutes included products from pigs. They no longer do, to the relief of many people.

After it became clear that the fat in mother's milk is particularly good for the development of the brain and the sight of a newborn baby, work began to add artificial omega-3 fatty acids to formula. Such formulas can already be found in stores, although long-term results are not yet available. These types of fatty acids are supposed to be particularly good for babies. With or without them, never before have we had such good artificial nutrition for babies. If your baby requires a substitute for your milk, be glad you live now!

The Advantages of Bottles

The disadvantages of bottle feeding are clear: the baby doesn't benefit from the special advantages of breast milk, and the mother and child don't experience the benefits of breastfeeding. But bottle feeding also has its advantages. You can see how much food your baby is taking and you don't have to wonder if it is hunger that is making your baby scream. Breast milk substitutes are relatively consistent. They don't vary depending on what you eat and drink or on whether you take medication or what time of day or night it is.

The father or others can also more easily help with bottle feeding. Some regard the ability to be away from the baby as an advantage. Nonetheless, experience shows that mothers who give bottles are usually with their newborn baby most of the time anyway. You will avoid problems that can occur with your breasts during milk production, such as mastitis or soreness. You may, however, have had a particularly tough time at the beginning, when it became clear that your baby was not going to be breastfed.

Preparing the Formula

Follow the instructions on the box carefully when making up the mixture. Too much powder will be too hard on the baby's tummy and too concentrated for the whole body. So don't be too generous no matter how well you wish your baby. If you use too little powder, the milk will be too thin and will not have enough nutritional value.

For the most part, tap water in the Western world is very clean and pure; even so, it should be boiled before it is mixed with the powder. Buy six to eight bottles so that you don't have to boil or sterilize them more than once a day. Boil the clean equipment for at least five minutes. While your baby is tiny, treat all equipment in this way.

Most parents think it's a good idea to make enough milk mixture for a whole day. It shouldn't be stored for much longer than this. The milk can be kept in the refrigerator for twenty-four hours—but ideally not in the refrigerator door, which is warmer. Ready-mixed milk spoils if kept for a long time at room temperature.

Some parents make one bottle at a time, according to need. This can be a good idea when you're traveling or where keeping things cool is difficult. Dry powder keeps well, and getting hold of boiled water is normally easy.

Put the water in the bottle first. You can also have a sterile bottle filled with newly boiled water, which you can keep for a few hours at room temperature. Put the exact amount of powder in the bottle. Put on the cover and the ring and shake well before putting on the nipple. Ideally, very small babies should have the milk at about body temperature. Warm the bottle in a pan of water after you have taken the nipple off. Test the temperature by dripping a few drops on the inside of your wrist. Be careful when heating milk in the microwave oven. It can become unevenly warm, with some areas scalding, even though the rest seems to be all right. Mix and shake well before giving it to your baby, and test the temperature carefully.

Turn the bottle upside down and see how quickly the milk comes out. Two to three drops per second are ideal. A hole that is too small makes it tiring to suck. A hole that is too large makes the milk run too quickly so that the baby doesn't get to satisfy its sucking needs.

Turn the ring back so that it sits properly on the bottle. A little air will then get into the bottle while the baby sucks, eliminating a vacuum, which can make the nipple compress, forcing the baby to suck harder and harder to get the milk out.

BOTTLE FEEDING

Stimulate your baby's reflexes by stroking your fingers a little over the baby's lips and the cheek nearest to you, before you give the baby the bottle. The baby's lips will start to move, the mouth will open, and a little searching will take place as your infant turns toward you following stimulation of the cheek. Your baby is getting ready to suck, and the digestive processes are starting to work. You could also drip a few drops of milk onto the mouth so that your baby recognizes the taste if it seems interested.

Hold the bottle at an angle so that the nipple is always full of milk, not air. If a vacuum causes the nipple to compress, turn the bottle a little in the baby's mouth so that air gets in. Take the bottle away as soon as it is empty.

Pauses in sucking must be permitted. Sucking and breathing at the same time can tire the baby. If the baby goes to sleep while feeding, you may want to take away the bottle and pick the baby up for a burp. Rub the back gently and pat the baby's bottom or back. Air tends to collect in the baby's stomach during bottle feeding, and this can give a false sense of fullness. After burping the baby, you can offer the bottle again. Always finish by burping the baby, however, to prevent bloating or a tummyache as the result of swallowed air. For the baby that holds onto the burp, try sitting the baby on your lap and gently bend it forward a bit at the hips.

MIXED FEEDING

Some mothers give both breast milk and formula. This can be tiring but allows mother and baby to experience some of the advantages of both. Don't start using a bottle as long as you hope to be able to breast-feed exclusively. Using a cup is better. If you clearly must continue to use supplements, give the baby the breast first and then top off with a bottle.

Mary Anne had no desire to breastfeed. Both her mother and her sister had used bottles for their babies. In this family, bottles were the tradition. Mary Anne also thought that her breasts would become ugly when breastfeeding. This is wrong. The main changes in the breasts occur during pregnancy. Most women are happy with their breasts after the breastfeeding period, providing they liked them before. The midwife in the maternity ward tried to get Mary Anne to change her mind, and she halfheartedly agreed to try. But she became sore and thought the baby screamed a lot. At home, her experienced relatives recommended using a bottle. Mary Anne held out for a while, but after she started giving every other meal with a bottle, she had less and less breast milk. When the baby was four weeks old, she stopped breastfeeding.

If you think about starting to use a bottle because you don't have enough milk yourself, remember that you can give small amounts of solids from four months; doing so may make a bottle unnecessary if you still have almost enough milk yourself. From six months, it's time to start giving solids anyway.

Forgive Us, for We Know What We Do

Finally, I would like to ask forgiveness from some of you. I know it seems hurtful when the media, health personnel, and WHO and UNICEF continually promote breastfeeding, with its many advantages, assisted by people like me.

I remember the surprise and sorrow when I had to give up on breastfeeding when my own first baby was six weeks old. I had thought that breastfeeding would be simple. Stopping was also a relief, though—and how he enjoyed his bottle! For me, having to give up turned into an incentive to work toward a better understanding of what went wrong.

Giving up feels even worse today when virtually everyone else is breastfeeding, in Norway, anyway. Mary Anne recently sent me a letter, having read the newspaper: "After I had my first baby, and to my great dismay, I had to start using bottles when the baby was about three weeks old. I have taken serious note of the stream of articles on breastfeeding. Without even looking for it, I feel I have been bombarded with information on all the dangers to which my baby will be exposed because I couldn't manage to breastfeed her. Even now, after four months, when I have more or less come to terms with things, and when I don't start crying every time I read one of these articles, it is still depressing."

The really sad thing about Mary Anne was that she didn't seem to have gotten enough good help. She was bitter about this, and I agree that she had a right to be. At the same time, I tried to explain to her in my reply that knowledge about the benefits of breast milk is one of the most important tools we have for motivating health personnel to become better at helping those who are struggling with breastfeeding. Mary Anne and I agreed that she should contact me before having her next baby; I'm pretty sure I can help her. In the meantime, I have asked her to enjoy her bottle-fed baby and say to herself firmly, "Remember, I am just as good a mother, even though I bottle fed my baby. There are many ways of giving both food and love!"

While feeding your baby with a bottle, make sure that:

- You hold the baby close to your warm body.

- The baby has skin-to-skin contact.

- The baby gets eye contact whenever it wants it.

- You talk to your baby.

Following are guidelines for a baby's food intake:

- A baby needs a total of around 5 ounces of milk per 2.2 pounds of body weight every twenty-four hours.

- Example 1: An 8.8-pound baby needs about 18-20 ounces of milk per day. If fed every four hours, this means six meals per day with 3 ounces of milk in the bottle.

- Example 2: A 13.2-pound baby needs 30 ounces per day. With six meals, this means 5 ounces of milk per bottle.

- Also, bottle-fed babies have varying appetites, and some need food more often. The amount per meal should then be reduced correspondingly.

To prepare the formula:

- Pour freshly boiled water into a sterilized measuring cup with a spout.

- Measure out the powder exactly, leveling off at the top of the measuring spoon with a knife.

- Add the powder to the water and stir with a clean spoon until it has dissolved.

- Pour the milk mixture straight into the bottle, possibly through a sterilized funnel.

- Put the nipple on the bottle, without letting it come in contact with the milk.

- Put on the cap, fasten the ring tightly, and put on the cover.

After feeding:

- Throw away any leftover heated milk.

- Rinse the bottle in cold water, pay extra attention to the nipples.

- Using a bottle brush, wash all parts in warm, soapy water.

- Rinse thoroughly.

- From time to time, rub coarse salt into the nipple and rinse well. Check that the holes are open; if not, use a large needle to open any that are clogged.

CHAPTER 17

. . .

Infant Development

The younger the baby, the less voluntary control that baby has over its movements. At the start, the muscle flexors are dominant. The baby lies with fists clenched, bending the arms and legs in toward the body just as was done in the womb.

REFLEXES

John was very proud of his healthy newborn son Trevor. He put his big index fingers into the small clenched fists and demonstrated this: "Look, he's holding himself up when I lift him." John was a doctor and knew about a newborn baby's reflexes. What he was showing was the grip reflex, which is so strong in many newborn babies that they can actually hang from their hands, quite similar to a baby chimpanzee, which clings tightly to its mother. "King of the monkeys!" John scolded his little son gently when he grabbed John's hairy chest and tugged hard.

John fooled his family and friends into believing that little Trevor was something unique—not the least by having his son "walk" as a newborn. The tiny soles of Trevor's feet were placed on a solid surface. The baby stretched his legs and put his weight on his feet. When John bent him over a little forward, he began to walk across the table.

Father and son had several tricks to perform. John held Trevor around his body, under the armpits, and stroked the soles of Trevor's feet against the edge of the table. The baby then lifted his feet and placed them on the table. This is the so-called location reflex. The same reflex is invoked when the backs of the hands are stimulated a little later in the child's development.

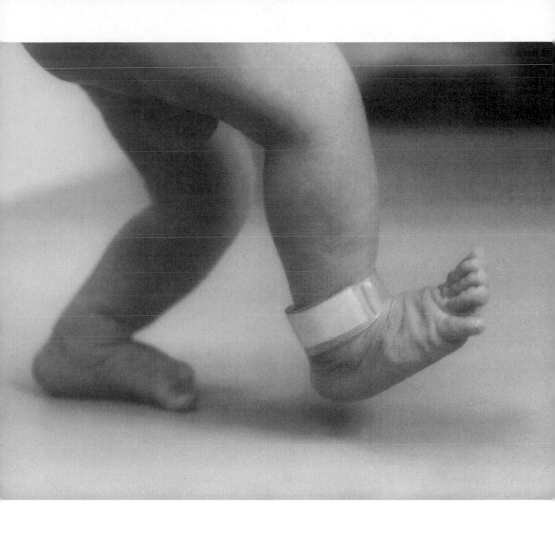

In truth, we were all child prodigies at the beginning. This has nothing to do with either intelligence or extraordinary physiology. Reflexes are automatic, and many even disappear over time. It's quite entertaining to know about some of them, though, and to admire them in your own baby.

The most important reflexes—if the newborn is to survive—are the search reflex (causing the mouth to turn toward whatever stimulates the cheeks), the sucking reflex (causing the baby to suck whenever something touches the roof of the mouth), and the reflex that enables the baby to move the hand toward the mouth. All of these reflexes are designed so that the baby can get hold of food. By three to four months of age, however, the gripping reflex of the hands has almost disappeared. Also disappearing at this time is the Moro reflex, which previously caused the baby to fling out its arms in fear if any support disappeared.

Physical Development

The same son of whom John was so proud definitely could not hold his head up for long periods as a newborn, but could lift it only in unsteady jerks. Trevor was developing at about the same rate as most other newborns. Eventually, the baby's control over his head increased, so that he could hold it steadily when he lay on his tummy at two months. When he saw his parents, his whole body became active. His mouth gaped, and he waved with his arms so that he looked like a seal using its flippers; at the same time, his legs stretched out, stiff with eagerness.

After three months, Trevor could lift not only his head but also his chest when he supported himself on his arms. When he lay on his tummy, he began to "swim" with his arms and his legs. He could manage to turn himself onto his back but could not turn back onto his tummy.

At around four months, Trevor could hold his head still in most positions, turn it, and follow everything intensely. He could rock on his stomach like a rocking horse, with his arms and legs up in the air. At about this time, he also started to use his grip consciously and would beam when he managed to hold a toy.

Then Trevor began to reach for things and to grasp smaller objects with his fingers, no longer with his whole hand. When he was about five months old, he managed to turn from his back onto his stomach, too, after a lot of practice. From time to time, he grabbed his own toes and fingered them with interest. The proud father thought it was fantastic when Trevor managed to suck his own big toe.

At around six months, Trevor could sit up with a bit of support, although he sometimes lost his balance or ended up with his chin between his knees. Now he lifted his head while lying on his back and considered his toes or his penis with satisfaction. He began to move toys from one hand to the other.

The family had to watch out because Trevor put everything he grasped into his mouth. In this way, he also began to taste the family's food. He chewed on dry crusts, splashed his hand in the jam, and smacked his lips with satisfaction. He was clearly indicating that he was ready for new tastes in addition to breast milk, as long as he could decide the menu. Things were not so good when he got mustard on his index finger or when he grabbed hold of the baby ointment and sucked on that with intense joy.

Although there are some variations, development more or less follows this regular pattern among healthy babies. Where premature babies are concerned, it is important to calculate their maturity from the day when they were due to be born (after a full-term pregnancy) to avoid worry. In contrast, babies who arrive late may appear very precocious. In early infancy, the time from conception counts most.

Training cannot speed the achievement of such milestones, but it is important for your baby to be stimulated and given the opportunities to develop at the right times. A baby who doesn't have something to reach for won't learn to grip. A baby not given the chance to try new tastes at around six months may refuse to do so later on. A baby not lain on its tummy to play won't develop strong neck and back muscles.

The teeth normally start appearing after about six months, but they may erupt much later or earlier. Some babies are even born with teeth.

THE SENSES

Feeding, and breast feeding in particular, leads to an intense combination of taste and smell. It's not surprising that a newborn baby turns toward the smell of milk and mother. Research has shown that newborn babies can distinguish between very different smells.

Touch is important for the baby's physical development. Babies who do not have skin-to-skin contact and tenderness do not develop normally, even if they have enough food and are otherwise well looked after. Baby apes who do not find a soft mother to cling to later don't manage to take care of their own firstborn babies very well. Yet after they have a chance to practice with their first baby, things go somewhat better for them if they have a second.

Most of us will instinctively cuddle the lovely little baby we are looking after. We stroke the body as we comfort and try to calm the infant. Many cultures have incorporated this into their systems for infant care and give newborn babies a massage every day. Books and courses on this are available.

I don't think it really matters how you stroke your baby as long as you do so gently and tenderly. Try it. What does your little one seem to like best? Are fingertips preferred—or big, warm hands? Are gentle strokes across the stomach best? A firm grip on the arms and legs? Stroking the back? Cuddling a slender neck, or a naked bottom? Maybe all of these? Most babies love this type of contact. Some may not like it so much, and try to ward it off, however. If this is the case, proceed with caution and try to interpret your baby's reaction.

Skin contact expresses and promotes love. It increases the hormone oxytocin, which has a calming effect and reduces anxiety. It affects the baby, who enjoys the experience and will later be able to give the same kind of contact as a result. Adults who have not experienced such tenderness transmitted through the skin may later react with suspicion and disgust. This may have consequences both for close adult relationships and for relationships with their own small children.

In the beginning, vision functions best at a distance of about 10 inches, approximately the distance to the mother's eyes when she is breastfeeding. The newborn baby focuses only briefly and then turns the head toward light. These newborns always choose to look at a face over anything else. They prefer to look at an oval shape with dots that represent eyes, nose, and mouth, rather than at an oval shape with just as many dots that don't represent anything. They look for eye contact but turn their eyes away when they have had enough. Respect these signals.

Babies tested when twelve hours old showed that they could recognize colors; they demonstrated this by looking longer at some colors (usually green and blue) than at others. After three to four weeks, babies fix their gaze on something moving about 4 inches to the side. At about three to four months, the vision of a baby is similar to that of an adult.

Hearing develops long before birth. Research has shown that babies recognize voices, songs, poetry, and stories that they heard in the womb. Yasmine was full of guilt and remorse because she had not sung to her unborn baby. This is nonsense, of course! The fetus is just as happy listening to all the things that her mother talks about throughout the pregnancy.

A newborn baby is frightened of loud noises and is comforted by soft voices. Early on, babies turn toward sounds that can be heard half a yard away. Eventually they begin to understand the significance of sounds. They may stop crying at the sound of approaching footsteps or be excited by sounds that indicate food. Many babies react with irritation to mechanical noise, from household equipment, for example, while others are calmed by the rhythmic sounds from a washing machine or dishwasher.

But most of all, babies like to listen to voices—especially to "baby talk," with simple expressions repeated in a high, light voice. They become quieter and more peaceful when they hear such sounds. After a few weeks, they start to express different moods using their own voice. Vigilant parents can distinguish between sounds that mean hunger, tiredness, and joy.

Psychological and Social Development

Newborn babies prefer to look at their mother's face and also prefer the known to the unknown. Eventually they look at anybody who talks to them and at mobiles and other dangling toys.

The baby's social smile appears around four to six weeks after the term date. This is of enormous significance. The person at whom the smile is directed looks back at the baby in astonishment, changes the tone of voice, and becomes cheerful and energetic in relation to the baby. Around three months, most babies smile and babble with joy whenever somebody talks to them. They wave their arms and legs and fix the other person with their gaze.

At about four months, babies learn to laugh out loud. They are fascinated at the sight of toys and show interest when they see the breast or a bottle. Increasingly babies at this age will turn toward a sound.

From five months onward, babies will normally look for something they have dropped or for a person moving away. Babies understand that things can be found even when they can no longer be seen. They smile at themselves in the mirror.

Memory develops gradually. The newborn can remember for six to eight hours. As a typical example, consider a baby who has had a bad experience while being breastfed, possibly feeling smothered. That baby, when picked up the next time to be put to the breast, may begin to cry. After a few weeks, babies can remember two days, and at three months of age, they remember more than four weeks—much longer than earlier believed.

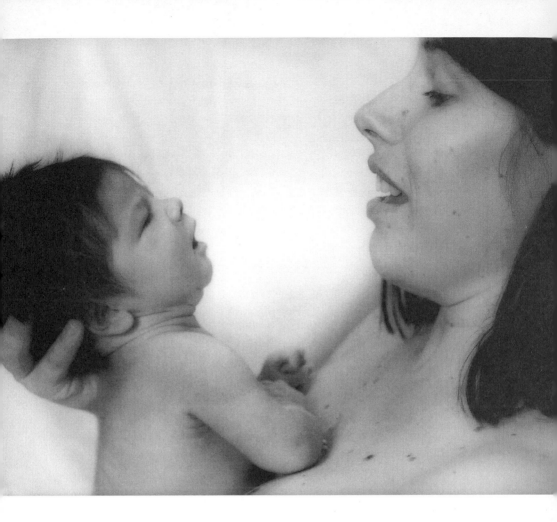

Temperament and personality vary considerably from one baby to another. Inherited characteristics and experiences in the womb and during birth all differ. Some newborn babies are robust, whereas others are delicate and irritable. Newborns studied by researchers and described as having a peaceful temperament generally appear to have a better relationship with their surroundings after a year than do babies described as being irritable and screaming in the days after birth.

Some babies love physical contact and will relax completely against an adult body, clearly enjoying themselves. Others struggle and wriggle when held and are much more difficult to comfort. Parenting these babies is a bit harder.

Boys have proved to be a little more demanding than girls. Although parents' attitudes toward boy and girl babies may be different, the extra demand probably has more to do with physical reasons. Still, adults have been shown to talk in a different way to a newborn dressed as a girl than to the same baby dressed as a boy. Requests for help with breastfeeding are more common when the baby is a boy, perhaps because the parents react with greater uncertainty to a more unsettled baby.

A mother's anxiety or depression is believed to affect the baby to some extent. Children of mothers who were depressed for a month after the birth, for example, usually find it more difficult to control their emotions later in life. The same can happen if the baby gets too little or far too much stimulation. The social network is also of great significance. Irritable babies become worse if the mother is isolated and is largely at home alone with the baby. Speak to a healthcare provider—who can help you with contacts—if you feel depressed or isolated.

Babies prefer to look at people rather than at anything else. They are born as social beings. Many newborn babies manage to imitate others. Some researchers observed two-week-old babies while the infants studied an adult's face. Although the researchers could see only the babies, they had no problem deciding whether the baby was imitating happiness, sadness, or surprise.

For the first six months, the baby is mostly interested in the closest person providing care, usually the mother. The baby will watch both father and mother, but the adult takes most of the initiative for communication. Some adults are very active—talking, playing, and laughing. Others are quiet and passive. In her doctoral dissertation, "The First Dialogue," Bjørg Røed Hansen concluded that the mother's attention, rather than her activities in relation to the baby, decided the infant's psychological development. Being aware of the baby is necessary for being able to understand the baby's signals. You do not need to entertain and stimulate the baby the whole time; you simply need to be present as much as possible, looking at and listening to your infant.

Because of innate reflexes, a newborn baby can:

- Grip and hold onto anything that touches the palms of the hands.

- Search for anything touching the cheek or mouth.

- Suck on anything touching the roof of the mouth.

- "Stand," "walk," and put down the feet.

- Fling arms out if the support beneath the baby suddenly gives way.

Milestones in physical development during the first six months:

- Two months: Babies hold head up steadily when lying on their front side.

- Three months: Babies can also hold chest up when lying on their stomach. Babies can turn onto their back.

- Four months: Babies consciously grip using the whole fist.

- Five months: Babies can grip small objects with their fingers. Babies can turn from back to stomach.

- Six months: Babies can sit with support. Babies can lift head when lying on their back. Babies can move objects from one hand to the other.

Remember that individual babies may vary significantly from these guidelines; they are only approximations.

Psychological and social development:

- From birth: Babies look at person talking to them.

- Four to eight weeks: First social smiles appear.

- Three months: Babies babble and smile at everyone. Babies can remember for several weeks.

- Four months: Babies laugh out loud and turn toward sound.

- Five months: Babies look for things they have dropped.

Pay attention to your baby: look, talk, listen, and answer.

. . .

CHAPTER 18

Why Is the Baby Crying?

Previously, a newborn baby's cry signaled the successful survival of birth. A baby who didn't cry was smacked, pinched, turned upside down, or dunked alternately in hot and cold water. Those waiting impatiently outside the delivery room were moved and relieved when they finally heard the baby cry. And it's true: the first cry is a reassuring signal that a living baby has been born and is managing to get air in and out of the lungs.

The newborn baby does not need to cry out, however. Nowadays we look at the newborn expectantly, and if breathing is well and color is good, we don't need to hear a cry. Baby mammals in general do not normally make loud noises the moment they are born. In fact, doing so would be unwise, because it would make others aware of the presence of a helpless little one.

Newborn human babies today have far less reason to cry out than they did a generation ago. In Norway at least, most babies are quickly put on their mother's stomach. This is both calming and stimulating. But all babies cry at some time, and the majority cry more than their parents have anticipated and much more than their parents would like.

Why does your baby cry? This is the newborn's only way of saying, "Here I am, I need you!" Crying is a way to connect with parents. Hunger is the most common cause, and this is the most usual interpretation. Breastfeeding gets off to a flying start because the baby is signaling again and again: "I want—I want—I want!"

Barbara interpreted the crying as hunger. She put her baby to her breast every time the crying began. A few days after the birth, her mother's milk came in in earnest. The baby's weight increased, and everything seemed to be going fine. After they came home from the hospital, however, the baby cried more and more, sometimes even right after being fed. He latched onto the breast eagerly every time it was offered but often let go of it quickly, belched, and was restless. The parents tried using a pacifier, but this didn't help much.

After a while, Barbara and Dave began to notice slight differences in the crying. Often it was less powerful, more complaining and calling. They tested this out and eventually discovered that this type of cry meant, "I'm lonely. I want someone to hold me, carry me, comfort me."

They also found that things worked best when Dave, the father, dealt with these cries. When Barbara picked up the little boy, he smelled milk and food and searched eagerly for her breast, even though he had just finished feeding. Then he became overfull and irritable, burped, got cross, and pushed away the breast in between sucking.

When they were reasonably certain that the baby was not crying of hunger, Dave put him over his shoulder or left him hanging over his arm and walked up and down while bending his knees a little. The baby lay quite still, looking, with a wide-awake expression. When Dave stopped, the crying started again.

"Spoiled," said the mother-in-law.

"Full, but lonely," said Barbara.

"He likes to go for a walk with his daddy," said Dave proudly. He maintained that, after three months, there were deep tracks in the hardwood floor and that together they had done several marathons.

"Good training," he said, while he stood and did hundreds of knee bends with his son over his shoulder, not just a little proud that he was the best at stopping this type of crying.

In a Finnish survey, about three-fourths of the mothers asked said that their babies often cried "calling" or "quietly." Most of the mothers felt that their baby's crying aroused a need in them to comfort the baby. About one-fourth of them thought that the baby cried "strongly," but only a few thought that the cry expressed "anger." Many felt that it had

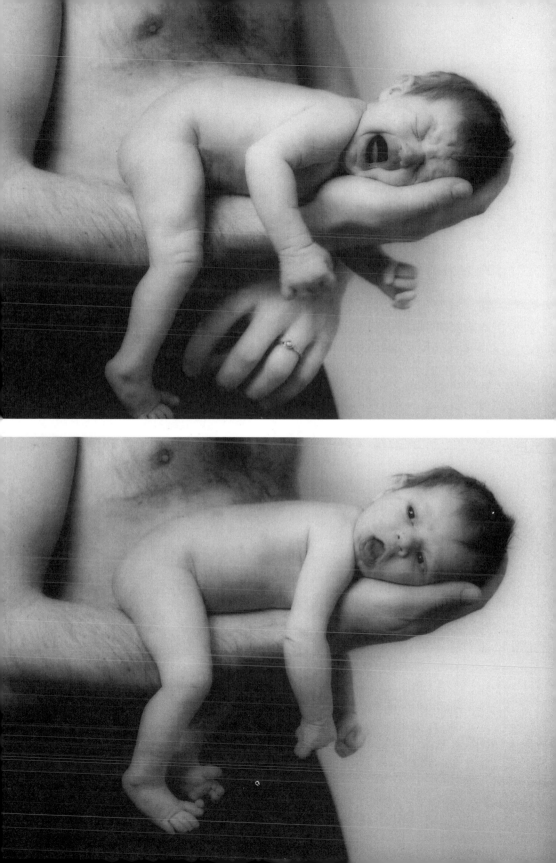

a "disturbing" or "irritating" effect, however. Some felt that the baby's cry was "frightening" or gave them a "feeling of failure."

Let the Baby Cry?

Can't you just let the baby lie there and cry? Yes, of course you can. He is hardly going to cry himself to death. A popular belief for some decades was that it was good for the baby to scream because it strengthened the lungs. This may be true, but what did this do to the baby itself? I have heard a psychologist say that a little child who sends out the strongest emergency signals possible but does not get a reply may later develop into a person who lacks basic trust and has trouble feeling that he is fully loved for himself. That doesn't sound unreasonable, does it?

Some professionals think that an infant who does not feel able to influence his or her own situation may grow up to be a passive individual who easily gives up. Maybe this is why a crying baby makes most of us feel that we simply have to do something. If so, this appears to make sense. In any case, it's impossible to spoil a baby in the first few months. Later on is another matter. If we look again to the animal kingdom, it is incredible how patient and self-sacrificing most animal mothers are with their offspring in the first few weeks. These same animal mothers become quite bossy later on.

Big Tummy Kitty and Little Tummy Kitty

Some babies cry because they eat too much. Once our cat had two kittens that looked exactly the same. The only thing that distinguished them was the way they ate. One pushed its way to the best teat, trampled the teat energetically with its tiny forepaws, and sucked strongly. When the kittens became bigger, this one nearly leaped into a full saucer of milk. In the beginning, our children distinguished the kittens from each other by feeling their little tummies after they had eaten. Big Tummy Kitty had a tummy as tight as a drum. His brother held back more when food was offered and was called Little Tummy Kitty.

Amy's little daughter seemed to be like Little Tummy Kitty. She had enough to eat, and her weight went up fine. But she cried and cried, and carrying and cuddling could seldom soothe her. Amy had learned it was best to offer both breasts at every feeding, and she always changed over to the second breast after about eight to ten minutes.

I advised her to try giving her daughter only one breast each time she fed. In return, the baby could suck as long as she wanted from that breast and would usually happily stay there for half an hour. From the first day of this regime, the baby changed her behavior and was much more peaceful.

The explanation was probably that this baby had a small stomach but a strong need to suck. When she was given both breasts, her stomach became full before her need to suck was satisfied. Her tummy did not have enough room for milk from both breasts at a time. It became distended and too full of the sugary foremilk. When she sucked on only one breast, however, her stomach became full enough, and then she continued sucking on the apparently empty breast. Amy thought that her baby did this for enjoyment, but she was wrong. In fact, the milk that the baby gets hold of when the breast is nearly empty is usually particularly rich and full of extra calories. When the baby sucks on a soft, more or less empty breast, fine droplets of fat are released into the milk, making cream. The baby swallows a small quantity but receives many calories. This gives the baby a feeling of being satisfied without the stomach becoming overfull.

Baby Patrick's situation was exactly the opposite. His tummy had a large capacity and he became irritated and impatient when the mother's milk tapered off from the first breast. Only after feeding from both breasts did he feel relatively full. Then he slowly enjoyed the cream from the last breast before he fell asleep, bursting and content.

If you have a baby who cries a lot quite soon after being breastfed, try these two methods to find out if your baby has a big tummy, which needs both breasts to feel full, or a small tummy, which has room only for milk from one breast. If you take note of the baby's signals, you might be able to solve the problem. Feeding on demand doesn't mean just giving the baby the breast when he wants it; it also means interpreting signals about when it is time to change breasts and when the baby perhaps just needs a little break from sucking.

Often a Little Tummy baby will take less per feeding but will need to be fed more often. All is well as long as everybody is satisfied.

This problem of babies' stomachs being overextended from too much foremilk without room for the fat-rich aftermilk is described in the prestigious medical periodical *The Lancet*. This Little Tummy condition is given as a common but rarely recognized reason for crying. Now you know the remedy.

"Change My Diaper!"

Some babies seem to cry because they are wet or have a dirty diaper. Dirty diapers should always be changed. Wet diapers, however, don't seem to irritate most babies particularly. A study showed that babies became calmer when they were changed, even if the same wet diaper was put back on again. On the whole, most babies don't mind being slightly damp, as long as they are warm and not sore. Maybe these babies simply enjoy being wrapped up? Or maybe they like to lie naked and sprawling?

The best way to avoid soreness is to use as little soap as possible and, ideally, to rinse the baby's bottom only under the tap or clean it with a little oil. Let the baby lie without diapers for a while, air-drying, before putting on a clean diaper. A bit of sunshine on a sore bottom for a little while can also be good. If the bottom does get sore, use a protective cream after airing before putting a diaper on again.

"Wrap Me Up!"

On several occasions, my husband and I have lived with a nomadic family with many young children in the Sahara. On our first visit, we jumped when we heard a soft sound from little heap of sand with a camel saddle over it. After a while, we took a peek under a carpet covering the camel's saddle. There lay the new baby, Mofta, just eleven days old, under several layers of rags. He was swaddled—wrapped up securely with a small strip of cloth—so that he looked like a shrimp. He wore no diaper—just a thin layer between him and the sand, which absorbed everything that came out. His conscientious mother carefully cleaned him with sand and rags among all the flies. Using signs, she indicated that he cried a lot less when he was bundled up like this.

As opposed to the baby who calms down when allowed to lie naked and sprawling is the baby who becomes unsettled in the limitless world outside the womb. A few years ago in Saint Petersburg, Russia, I saw many newborn babies, all swaddled, with their arms and legs straight, just as we used to swaddle babies in Norway some generations ago. That's the way it was supposed to be; babies were much more peaceful then.

Unfortunately, swaddled babies have been shown to have a greater tendency to lung problems, so the practice is not recommended. Newborn babies also need to be able to lie in the frog position, a position that is natural for them and promotes the development of good, deep hip sockets.

However, if your baby is restless and flailing and appears to be terrified by his or her own movements, however, you can try wrapping the baby quite tightly in a baby blanket. Some babies calm down very well when wrapped like this. Maybe they are missing the cramped conditions of their mother's womb and need time to get used to plenty of room and lots of opportunities to move. Wrapping like this can also help babies who flail about so much with their hands that they lose their grip on the breast, or it can be helpful if you are trying to feed an infant from a cup.

All babies cry, and most cry more than their parents had anticipated. They normally cry for half an hour up to four hours per day. This crying often increases at the age of two weeks and approaches a maximum at around six weeks. Then it normally decreases and becomes more rare after twelve weeks. Some babies have few but long-lasting crying bouts, while others cry every hour of the day, luckily usually for short periods only. Babies tend to cry most in the evenings and before they are fed but only a little in the morning.

COLIC

About every fifth baby under the age of three months cries for more than three hours per day for at least three days per week. This is often called colic. These babies pull their legs up under them, become red in the face, and appear to be suffering. Colic is more common among firstborn babies. Even though it is quite common, we still don't know the cause. Many theories exist: it may be caused by an upset digestive system and a lot of air; by an immature nervous system; by hypersensitivity to cow's milk; by allergies; by acidic stomach contents that come up into the esophagus, and result in pain; by disturbances in the mother-baby relationship; by problems with the neck following the birth, and so on.

All treatments appear to have good short-term results because colic is a condition that is self-healing. In the meantime, you find yourself with an apparently desperately uncomfortable baby, wanting to help that baby so much, often suffering yourself.

This is what it was like for Joseph's parents. He cried and cried, pulled his legs up under him, farted, curled up, and screamed. Patting him and carrying him helped only a little. One day his parents found that he lay completely still when put in his baby seat on top of the spinning washing machine—but they couldn't keep that up the whole time. He was often calmer when they went for a drive in the car or when he was out in his stroller.

Joseph's granny had some success calming him when she made some solid bumps with a rug, brought his stroller inside, and pushed it back and forth across the bumps. His parents acquired a baby rocker, which made his whole crib vibrate. All of this helped—for a while. Then he would return to crying, just the same as before.

Joseph's family was advised to try having a chiropractor manipulate Joseph's neck. A neighbor's child had benefited from this. However, the family did not want to expose Joseph's slender little neck to manipulation. Also, the treatment had worked for the neighbor's child only after six weeks. By then, the baby had been exactly three months old, which is just the age when colic usually disappears anyway.

Joseph screamed and screamed. His family took him to the doctor, but nothing seemed to be wrong. He grew and was content, apart from the screaming fits. The family knew that colic was more common in firstborn babies and were worried that they weren't dealing with it in the right way. Initially, his parents became jealous when others with more experience managed to quiet their baby. They soon became experts themselves, however, and were the best at getting Joseph to calm down.

They tried holding him with his head up high when he fed, so that he could more easily burp up any air that he swallowed. Health center personnel told them that the advertised pharmaceutical remedies to prevent the formation of gas in the gut had not been proven to have any effect. Tiny quantities of sugar water might have a calming effect, however. They tried that. They were advised to dissolve 1 tablespoon of sugar in ½ cup of boiled water. This tasted good and sweet. Joseph was given just ⅓ teaspoon when the crying was at its worst. This helped, and he became more settled. As a rule, the effect lasted from half an hour to two hours. The sugar water did not eliminate the reason for Joseph's crying, however, and his parents did not want to continue giving him sugar at a time in his life when he really should be having just breast milk.

Finally, Joseph's mother was advised to cut out all dairy products for three days herself. She wasn't to drink milk, eat cheese, or make food using milk. This was a real challenge. After only one day, though, Joseph seemed to scream less. Could the problem really have been in the cow's milk proteins that had gone into her milk? After three days, his mother started using dairy products again. Joseph's crying became worse. A few days later, she was prepared to cut out all dairy products for a while, and Joseph became much better. He continued to cry some, but the situation was much more livable.

Tests show that around one-third of all breastfed babies with colic improve if their mother avoids dairy products. If she does this, however, she must ensure that she has a properly balanced diet without milk. She can get calcium, for example, by eating a lot of green vegetables and fiber-rich food, but she could also take calcium tablets. Sesame seeds, which can be used in bread, cereal mixes, and cakes, contain particularly large quantities of calcium. When the baby gets older, she could try using dairy products again.

All of the different advice tried by Joseph's parents to calm him has been shown to have some effect. And while they were working on the problem, time went by. Colic becomes rarer after the age of three months.

In cultures where mothers carry their babies with them all the time, you seldom hear a baby crying. A young African woman lived with us for a few weeks just after she had her baby at my hospital. She had come to Norway with nothing but her return ticket because she was afraid to give birth in her homeland after her first baby had died there during birth. She had no medical insurance, and because staying in a Norwegian hospital is expensive, I brought her home with me once the baby was twenty-four hours old.

My family and I were surprised when we got home from work or school every day and she would hand the baby over to us and go to have a shower.

"Why don't you do that during the day when you've got the house to yourself?" I asked her, impatient to start dinner.

"You mean I should leave the baby all on his own?" she asked, shocked. In her culture, apparently, no one ever leaves a newborn baby alone, not even in the next room. The baby is always in someone's arms until old enough to be fastened to the mother's back.

A woman from another poor country told me of a standard cure used in her village whenever a baby cried inconsolably. The baby would be fastened onto her back and she would go to work in the fields with a hoe. The energetic, monotonous, rhythmic movements—and maybe the rocking motion, up and down, with the head and bottom uppermost alternately—almost always had good results, providing that the baby wasn't ill. If you don't have a cradle, you could try rocking the baby in your arms.

Most babies enjoy bodily contact and being carried. Good baby slings can be purchased on the market. In the first few weeks, the baby should normally be carried on your front, so you can observe its face and support the head. The problem is that a baby who is not used to being fastened to an adult body may not always be happy in this position. Practice using a sling when the baby is peaceful and content.

Some babies calm down after a massage, a technique used in many countries, such as India. Books about baby massage are available to help you learn: the most important thing is to use a warm, firm stroking movement across the skin. Carefully massaging the stomach to help the contents of the colon toward the rectum has a soothing effect on some babies. Begin above the right groin with gentle stroking upward movements toward the diaphragm; move across the stomach toward the baby's left and then down the left side. Some also maintain that acupuncture and acupressure—pressure on the acupuncture points—can help, but more research is needed.

The Baby Is Tired

Some babies seem to need to cry when tired and must be allowed to do so for a while before they fall sleep, without being picked up and offered food or another clean diaper. Allowing the baby this short period of crying is quite different from letting the baby scream for hours.

Failure as a Mother?

In the Finnish study about crying among newborn babies, almost one-fifth of the 4,556 mothers said that they had needed and wished for more help and support when their baby cried. These mothers found the baby's crying to be particularly piercing, loud, and complaining. They became irritable and also felt that they were poor mothers.

All of these are common and legitimate feelings. I myself used to have nightmares in which I put my screaming firstborn son into the washing machine and watched him go round and round without hearing anything other than the quiet sounds of washing. If you have feelings of which you are ashamed, you need help and support. If the baby's father is not around, extend your search. If family, friends, or neighbors can't help, let your doctor know that things are getting to be a bit too much for you. One solution might be to pay a teenager to take the baby out in the stroller after school for a while.

In any case, ask for help. Remember, you are not a failure! At this time in your life, you should have been surrounded by experienced people who were fond of you, loved your baby, and would be glad to help you out. A study of a primitive, nomadic tribe showed that women who have just given birth never choose to be alone; they always keep within earshot of the tribe. These new mothers do not participate in activities or discussions but sit passively with the others, largely preoccupied with their baby. If the mother needs rest or can't quiet the baby, one of the other women takes over for a little while.

It can be helpful to know that boys cry a bit more than girls and seem to be a bit more irritable. Babies who have been through a particularly difficult birth also cry more. Cries from premature, sick, or disabled babies are often felt to be especially irritating and piercing. Otherwise, you will notice that the cry changes character if your baby is ill. This may have to do with stomachache, earache, fever, or any of a lot of other things. When a mother says that her baby is acting differently—and not least, that the baby is crying in a different way than normal—we should listen to her and take her seriously.

The Newfound Peace and Quiet

One big change over the last decade in maternity wards is that they have become so quiet. Crying babies are seldom heard because most babies are rooming-in with their mothers and are content to be there. Chicks that get to be around their mother seldom cheep. In incubators on chicken farms, in contrast, the chicks cheep desperately, all the time. The same applies to little lambs out in the pastureland. They *baa* intensely the moment they discover that they have come away from the ewe. Otherwise, they are quite quiet. Perhaps much of the crying of human babies has to do with our civilization's strange custom of leaving babies alone before they are ready for it.

If the baby's crying seems to be food related, try the following:

- Feed the baby as often as wanted.

- Check to see if the baby is putting on weight.

- See whether the baby settles better after one or two breasts.

- Allow the baby to suck the aftermilk, which is rich in fat.

- Let someone other than you try to comfort the baby if the baby has been fed.

- Remove all dairy products from your diet for one week.

- If this works, try dairy products in your diet again.

- If the problem gets worse, cut dairy products out of your diet for a longer period.

If the baby cries a lot, you can also try the following:

- Carry, rock, stroke, and sing to the baby.

- Change the baby's position; place upright over your shoulder.

- Pat the baby's back or bottom from below.

- Put the baby on the stomach over a strong arm or thigh.

- Gently rock the baby up and down with the head and bottom uppermost alternately.

- Allow the baby to lie naked and sprawling.

- Give the baby a bath.

- Massage the baby.

- Wrap the baby in a baby blanket.

- Take the baby to the doctor to rule out illness.

- Give the baby ⅓ teaspoon of sugar water, several times if necessary.

- See if the baby calms down with a pacifier, but use it within reason.

- Ask for some help if you're tired, depressed, or irritable.

- Check whether the baby needs a bit of time to cry him- or herself to sleep.

- Remind yourself that the worst is usually over after six to twelve weeks.

- Expose the baby to strong rhythmic movements.

- Try car rides, baby rockers, or a stroller ride over bumps.

CHAPTER 19

· · ·

Those Exhausting Nights

Are you exhausted? No wonder. Never before has anyone demanded that you be awake for large parts of the night and then get up and be ready for action the following day. Not long ago, you took for granted that wild late-night parties would be followed by late, sleepy mornings.

Most of us don't function well when we lack sleep. In fact, sometimes people are kept awake as a form of torture. You can break down and even become totally confused due to lack of sleep. But a brand-new mother must put up with having her sleep broken night after night. At the same time, she must make the most of her days as she gets to know her baby; she must learn all about breastfeeding and child care and cope with the changes in her body following childbirth. Through all of this, she is supposed to radiate happiness.

EXCITED AFTER THE BIRTH

On a recent doctor's rounds in the maternity ward with some medical students, Michelle told us, "I gave birth at nine o'clock at night. When the two postpartum hours in the delivery room were over, we were taken up to the maternity ward. The baby was left in the nursery because the staff were going to look after him for the first night, and I was put in a room with several other mothers, who were sleeping. I was completely worn out after two exhausting days. But I couldn't sleep. I was so excited. I was happy and laughing to myself. Burning with energy. I wanted to shout out that I had given birth, had produced a wonderful baby who liked being with me and who had sucked at my breasts. I'd show them, just as soon as the

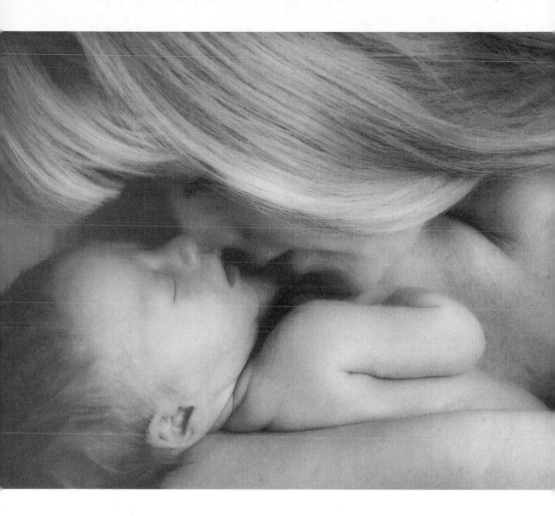

staff had finished looking after him. But after a while the excitement wore off. I was sad, irritated. I thought it was stupid that Steve had to go home. We should have had the chance to talk through the birth that we had just shared. I longed for my baby intensely. I don't think I slept all night. I wondered if they were looking after him as well as I would because I was his mother. And I was wondering if he was screaming. I even shed a few tears. I was missing my own mother."

So many mothers tell a similar story. If you're reading this before you give birth, and if you give birth in the evening, remember Michelle's experience. Ask if your bed can be put out in the corridor if you can't stay in the delivery room. Anything is better than being separated from your baby and being taken into a room where everyone else is asleep when you are wide awake and excited. This is really the time to rejoice, boast, complain, get to know your baby, and share things. It's not a time to fall asleep as though nothing had happened—not for the majority of us, anyway.

The staff want to observe your baby at regular intervals during the first night because a baby may develop problems—with breathing, for example—even when everything seemed fine right after the birth. A heart problem may make itself known in this way. Normally, though, the nurses can observe enough simply by regularly coming in to check on you and your baby.

Should You Be Rooming with Your Newborn?

In the maternity ward, try to have your baby with you during the night, at least after a while. Of course, both the waking up and the being half asleep while constantly aware of the new life entrusted to you are tiring. A tiny movement, a little sniffle, and you're awake. But most babies settle happily next to their mother, at least when they suckle from her, even before any real milk comes in.

All of our hormones have daily fluctuations. Your body produces prolactin—the hormone that is so important for regulating the amount of milk at the beginning—in particularly large quantities when you breastfeed at night. Not only do you and your baby benefit from the calming, sleep-inducing effect of this hormone, but the high level of prolactin also promotes breastfeeding the following day. In several studies mothers have been asked to evaluate their tiredness when they left the maternity ward. The studies showed that most were tired. Those who had not had their baby in with them at night were just as tired as those who had chosen to sleep with their baby. Basically, having a new baby is exhausting—whether the baby remains at your side or not!

Days and Nights Run into Each Other

Obviously you feel tired, especially if you don't even feel a rush of pleasure when the baby snuggles close to you. Some babies just don't settle, whatever you do. This is how it was for Joan. She is a gentle and experienced mother. But her second baby, Michael, screamed inconsolably from the first day, both in the hospital and when they came home. Thomas, her husband, carried the little guy and rocked him, rocked him and carried him. Joan had plenty of milk and was calm enough not to worry too much. Not until he was six weeks old did Michael start to settle. Today he is the sweetest little boy, gentle and trusting. Nobody ever did figure out why he screamed. He got optimal care in every way. Sometimes that's just the way it is. It was a good thing that he was not born to nervous first-time parents.

People who have unsettled babies need to get help. In hospitals designated as "Baby-Friendly," the staff tip-toe around at night and listen at the doors. They offer to look after a baby who will not settle down with the mother and bring back the baby after a while to be breastfed. The choice to accept this service is yours—but remember, you must sleep a little to avoid becoming totally exhausted.

Erin stopped by when her baby was two weeks old. She was totally exhausted from waking up nights and frightened because she hated the sound of her baby crying. "He is so demanding," she complained. And little Tim asked for a lot—an awful lot, but no more than he was entitled to. He really needed his Mommy. All the time, night and day, at the beginning. He didn't know that Erin was so terribly tired. He didn't realize when he started to cry again at midnight that Mommy had just gone to sleep after one single hour of adult company with Daddy. He was merely indicating his needs when they occurred. It was up to his parents to satisfy those needs. Like all newborns, Tim was used to constant warmth, company, and food from his time in the womb. Now he was gradually going to have to get used to managing at times without all of those things.

Actually, Tim was really most awake during the night, Erin said. She heard from me: "Let him gradually learn to distinguish between day and night. When he wakes up at night, make as little fuss as possible. No lights, no lively conversation, or sudden movements. Don't change his diaper if he is just wet. Just feed him and then put him down gently. Pick him up and soothe him if necessary, but otherwise, give minimal stimulation."

NIGHT FEEDINGS

A while later, Erin recalled again: "Your advice helped a bit. He settles down fine after he's been fed at night. But he is still waking up several times and wants to be fed, even though I know he's had plenty." I told her about a study that showed that some babies have to learn to accept a bit more time between feedings. For this to happen, the baby can be comforted in ways other than through feeding, so that the gap between night feedings gradually increases. Erin tried this. After a couple of months, Tim was waking up only twice per night on average, and Erin felt she could live with that.

Most breastfed babies need feeding at night, at least during the first six months, and many go on requesting these nighttime feedings for much longer. Because breast milk is so easily digested, the body has already fully utilized it after a few hours. Also, it doesn't help the breasts to be left for a whole night without being emptied. They become overfull and interpret this as a sign that production must be reduced. You may wake up with an uncomfortably full feeling after a peaceful night's sleep, and this often means that you will have less milk later in the day.

DREAMING OF A WHOLE NIGHT'S SLEEP

Nonetheless, most parents dream of the baby sleeping through the night as soon as possible. They see this as a goal, a victory! Is it really a victory? Maybe not, if achieving this means that the helpless newborn will lie there crying until sleep comes with exhaustion. This is different from the overtired baby who needs to cry for a while before calming down.

In many of the letters I receive, I find more or less the same sentence again and again: "Feeding the baby at night seems to be more of a problem for my mother-in-law/my mother/the health adviser than it is for me. It's these people who say now it's got to stop." Is something wrong with these expectations?

As a young mother, I also fell into the hands of these rational experts. "Let him cry," they said about my first baby. His cot was in a separate room. I had to be kept back in bed while the poor little fellow screamed and screamed. Then it suddenly became quiet. My baby lay there, red faced and swollen, after tossing about so fiercely that his head was down at the end of his crib.

With my second son, the breastfeeding was going well. But the health adviser thought I should stop feeding him at night after a few months. "Let him cry," she said. It was rather tempting to have a peaceful night. We put the baby's crib at the far end of our flat, where it was harder for us to hear him. He cried and cried. I sat by his crib with tears running down my cheeks. He was desperate. He couldn't understand what had happened to his soft, warm mother who always used to come to him. After an hour, I gave up and picked up the shaking little bundle. I have always regretted that night.

My third baby came many years and plenty of experience later. She stayed right next to my body right from the start—slept in our bed or lay in a cradle right next to us. She never cried without being comforted. She was always surrounded by loving people and was always put to the breast when necessary. This third child was incredibly peaceful, contented as she grew up. Was it just a coincidence? Perhaps—but an awful lot of mothers tell a similar story.

Tips for Quieter Nights

Don't let anybody else decide whether you should grit your teeth and put up with your baby crying without responding. Be with your baby as much as possible. Different sleeping remedies have been recommended for babies. Be skeptical. Think of all the strange, authoritarian rules used to separate mothers and babies throughout the ages. Don't do anything that goes against what you feel is best, your wish to meet your baby's needs at almost any price.

You will hear a lot of good advice and can try it out to get your baby to sleep more at night. Not only adults but also babies sleep better after getting a good dose of daylight every day. Recent light research indicates that babies establish a night and day rhythm more quickly and begin to sleep more regularly if they have been outside for a good while every day. This effect probably has something to do with the sleep-inducing hormone melatonin, which is created in the brain. Melatonin cannot be stored. A daily dose of daylight is necessary for its production. This is why many people in the north of Norway sleep badly during the dark periods of winter.

Another piece of advice is not to let your baby fall asleep before being put to bed. If you put an awake but full and happy baby to bed, the baby is more likely to develop the ability to go to sleep on his or her own peacefully.

During the first six to eight weeks, I advise you to let the baby feed whenever he wants to, at all hours of the day and night. During the night, talk as little as possible, make sure the room is half dark, and don't change a wet diaper. On average, babies sleep around sixteen hours out of every twenty-four in this period, but with large individual variations. If your baby tends to wake up a short time after you have gone to sleep, it's perfectly all right to waken the sleepy baby for breastfeeding before you yourself go to bed. Most babies will be more than happy to be fed.

At some time after six weeks, your baby's time awake will increase. At around twelve weeks, the baby will usually change the sleeping-waking pattern, sleeping less during the day and more at night. This change obviously occurs over a long time. Try to wait a bit before picking up the baby at night. Stretch out your hand to stroke him; rock him if he is restless. The baby may go back to sleep again for a while without being fed. Video filming throughout the whole night shows that babies are awake far more often than their mothers would believe. At the age of two months, most still wake their parents between midnight and five o'clock in the morning. At about nine months, only 20 percent wake their parents during this time. Even though babies don't sleep the whole night at this age, they manage better to go back to sleep by themselves. Firstborn babies are more awake than subsequent children.

You Must Get Enough Sleep

In spite of your baby, you must get some sleep when you are worn out.

Grace was choking with tears. Her pretty fair hair was lank and uncombed, her blue eyes red rimmed. "I think life is just horrible. I'm a total mess, and I'm so tired. Anthony gives our baby girl a bottle some nights so that I can get some sleep. But I wake up anyway. Besides, I can also feel my breasts bursting with milk."

We went through the last twenty-four hours together while Grace searched for times when she could have had a nap but hadn't done so. "After the morning's first diaper change and feed, I am really very tired. But I usually have breakfast with Anthony. It's nice to have a little adult company before he goes to work. Maybe I should take a nap then? He could look after her and get her back to sleep before he leaves.

"During the day, I get really lonely. I tend to talk on the telephone while the baby sleeps, and I get a bit done in the house. I suppose I could try and sleep then. And then there are the evenings. We normally stay up until around midnight or one o'clock in the morning. These are the best times for us. But one evening I fell asleep while I was feeding the baby around ten o'clock and slept right through until she needed changing. Then I noticed that I felt much better the next day. Maybe I need to give up our cozy evenings in order to feel better during the day?"

I thought this sounded sensible and asked how Grace slept at night between feedings. "Pretty well," she said. "I get very sleepy when I breastfeed. Then I wake up again when I have to get up and change the baby's diaper and put her back in her own bed. Then it often takes a while before I fall asleep again."

When Grace stopped changing diapers at night except when they were dirty, and when she put the baby's crib right next to her double bed, she no longer had to get up, and she went back to sleep more quickly again herself. Grace was highly satisfied that she had found the solution herself. After a while, she felt that the tiredness was starting to go, and she began to stay up a little later in the evenings again.

Less Contact During the Day, Greater Demands at Night

Things went really well for Grace, with increasingly more peaceful nights, until her baby was ten months old. Then Grace called me. "It has all gone crazy again," she groaned. "She wakes me up several times during the night, and all my energy is disappearing. She will only let me cuddle her, even though Anthony is at home on leave now." What had happened? Well, Grace had started to work again. This is something that many mothers experience. The content and happy baby, now eating porridge and dinner in addition to breast milk, suddenly starts behaving like a little breast-only baby again—demanding and unsettled and always wanting to be fed, especially at night.

Grace found the answer when she realized what was happening. "She's missing me. Of course, she was used to being with me. Suddenly we disappear for most of the day, both me and my boobs. So she is making the most of the hours when she knows where I am, mainly in bed next to her.

"But we worked out what to do. I used my paid time off for breastfeeding to start work an hour later in the morning. [In addition to the ten to twelve months of paid maternity leave, Norwegian women also get one hour off per day for breastfeeding if they choose to go back to work sooner, e.g., after six months.] Then we began the day with a long cuddling and suckling period. I didn't use the breast pump at work, because she already ate so many other types of food and was breastfed often during my time off. When I came home, we delayed our own dinner until later, and I would lie down, with something to munch on, and just let her feed as long as she wanted to. As a rule, we would both fall asleep after a while, and this was lovely after a busy day at work. When she realized that there was just as much mommy to be had in total, our nights became quieter again after a while. She and Anthony had a good time together during the day. In fact, he was better at giving her other food and drinks from a cup than I was, so in the end, we both became experts in our own areas."

Both common sense and research show that there is a time for immediate satisfaction and a time for learning to postpone it a bit. Clear examples of this can be found in the animal kingdom. The bitch, for example, is a loving, self-sacrificing mother, tolerating everything, until one day she suddenly snaps at the puppy who is trying to push past her to get to the dish of food. Now the puppy is big enough to understand rank order! Or think about the mother bear, fiercely defending her young, staying close to them day and night to feed them and teach them. One fine day, the time is right. The mother bear chases her young up a tree and leaves forever. Animals know instinctively when their young can manage.

The human baby is helpless for so long, and human life is so complicated, that these things clearly are not instinctive for us. In any case, our big, active brains get in the way of instinct. Maybe we should try harder to be a little more like other mammals during the first period following birth. Perhaps we should rest with our newborn offspring day and night, except when we have to get food and do the most necessary things.

Try to Enjoy the Baby, Too

Despite being so tired, perhaps you could also manage to enjoy the nights with your baby. Enjoy the feeling that the two of you are a little island in a sea of humanity. Enjoy the warm, restless little body, so intensely full of life. Enjoy the quiet nighttime when your baby finally settles down and peace reigns as you both gradually slip off to sleep.

Never again will you be so much in demand, so totally loved, so absolutely necessary for somebody. Later in life, you will have nights when you miss this closeness terribly, when big children wriggle impatiently away from your loving arms and no longer want a goodnight cuddle; when your teenager is out nights, and you are out of your mind with worry; when the nest is empty of children, and you suddenly realize that they all went far too fast, those golden years. So work on things now. Acknowledge that these nights with your baby are also positive—if you can.

Learn to sleep when you can:

- In the morning when your husband gets up and can look after the baby.

- During the day when the baby sleeps.

- In the afternoon, if somebody can look after your baby or take your baby out in the stroller.

- In the evening, going to bed earlier instead of staying up.

- On odd nights when someone else takes care of your baby and you need only do the feeding.

For more peaceful nights:

- Create a difference between day and night, with low lights and sounds at night.

- Don't change your baby's diaper if it is just damp.

- Give your baby a good daily dose of daylight and fresh air to help with sleep.

- Feed your baby right before you go to bed.

- Let your baby sleep close to you so you don't have to get up.

- Fall asleep together at the start while feeding at night.

- Gradually let the baby lie for a little while before feeding.

- Know that changes in routine can lead to extra demands.

- Prevent extra demands by offering extra contact and breastfeeding during the day.

· · ·

CHAPTER 20

What About My Body?
Exercise, Sex, and Contraception

Weeks and months go by after the birth. The first, acute changes of the postnatal period are over. Breastfeeding is going well. You have gotten used to the demanding little person always wanting your body. Still, more time must pass before you feel as you did before you were pregnant.

"My Stomach Is Still Too Big"

Does your stomach still stick out? Were you really upset when you met your neighbor the other day and she asked you when the baby was due?

If your stomach is ever going to be allowed to stick out, it might as well be before and after delivery. If you can cope with this, that's fine. If you can't manage it, or if your husband is wondering when you will start looking like your old self again, you might want to look back to the old days. Then, the new mother was commonly bound, with long wide strips of stiff material fastened around her stomach. After that went out of fashion, woman were expected to use their muscles to pull in their stomach. That practice is OK, as long as it works. The stomach probably has a special ability to pull itself together after childbirth; when the womb contracts, your digestive system starts to work properly again, and the extra fluid disappears. Many women require time, however, for the stomach muscles to get back into shape. Meantime, if you allow your stomach to droop for weeks or months, you may miss out on a golden opportunity. Your body will not be able to use this important time for physiological shrinking. So it might be sensible to support your stomach for a while, perhaps by using a soft, elastic girdle that is rolled on, elasticized trousers with a high waist, or a wide scarf. Some women claim that they have benefited greatly from this type of support. Just make sure that whatever you use feels comfortable.

Stopping Your Breasts from Sagging

It is possible to do the same with your breasts when you start weaning your baby. If you haven't used a bra before, doing so might be sensible now. As you produce less and less milk, you can use a support bra in smaller sizes. In the old days, the final weaning often took place in conjunction with binding the breasts, which stops the milk production. At the same time, the connective tissue (the firm part of the breast) shrinks and becomes shorter, preventing the breast from drooping. Remember, though, that pregnancy itself causes the greatest changes in the breasts. Most women have more mature but just as pretty breasts after pregnancy and breastfeeding. Women who are very thin may lose the fatty tissue in the breast as well. (It is largely fat that distinguishes between big and small breasts.) Others put on so much weight during pregnancy that they too are dissatisfied with their breasts afterward.

Dieting

Don't try to actively lose weight during the breastfeeding period. If you still have some extra pounds once the baby is born, that's fine. These are extra reserves of energy for breastfeeding, nature's way of allowing pregnant women to store up fat as soon as they have access to plenty of food. This is particularly necessary in the many countries where nobody knows whether there will be food for the mother after the baby is born. Even in countries such as Norway and the United States, you may need a layer of fat at times. You may be ill and unable to eat—or you may be so busy and stressed that you forget to eat or do not benefit from the food.

Modern research shows that the majority of women who exclusively breastfeed past three to four months soon begin to use up this extra layer. Then the fat slides off the thighs and the bottom, areas that are often difficult to slim down otherwise.

You should not start dieting during the breastfeeding period because your body has stored a number of environmental toxins in your fatty tissues during your long life. If the old layer of fatty tissue is broken down as a result of too much dieting, more of the environmental toxins will be excreted in your milk. Measurements have shown that the level of environmental toxins (such as PCB) in the mother's milk is higher for the first baby than for later babies. That level is also lower in vegetarians than in people who eat all types of food from higher up the food chain, including fish from polluted waters and meat. Your baby is going to live in a polluted world. Toxins are everywhere, even in cow's milk and baby food. Nonetheless, limiting these as much as possible when starting your baby in life is probably sensible.

Varicose Veins

Did you develop varicose veins while you were pregnant? If so, increased pressure in the abdominal cavity and the relaxed walls of the veins may have caused this. Take the chance to tighten up your legs as well. Never stand when you can sit; never sit when you can lie down. If you have to stand for long periods, use the muscles in your legs to pump your blood upward toward your heart. Bounce up and down on your toes again and again. Tighten and relax your legs and thighs. If your varicose veins or the swelling are bad, start the day by putting on elastic stockings or tights before you even get up in the morning. Put your legs up whenever you are relaxing. Resting on the sofa with your legs up against the wall can work wonders. It is even more important that you follow this advice while you are pregnant and can possibly prevent this problem from occurring in the first place.

Pelvic Pain

Some women suffer from the undefined problem of deep pain in the pelvis even after delivery. If walking or turning over in bed is painful, for example, you should get treatment, ideally from a physical therapist with special knowledge in this area. Ask at your health center. In some areas, women with pelvic pain get together and exercise in a swimming pool with particularly warm water.

Postnatal Exercise

Eventually it might be a good idea to start going to a postnatal gym or to do "mother and baby" exercises. Many gyms arrange special classes for women who have recently had a baby. Ask at your health center. As well as getting exercise through these activities, it's often good to meet others in the same situation. Usually you take your baby with you, and the baby can join in the exercises if awake. It's good to exercise your stomach muscles with your baby lying on your breasts or to do knee bends with your baby in your arms. Most babies enjoy their mother's body movements. You should not start exercising too hard too soon in general, although you can exercise your stomach muscles right away. In the beginning, just lift your head and look at your legs, or press your spine against the mattress so that your stomach becomes hard; then maintain that position for a little while. Or pull your stomach in as if you were going to put on a tight skirt and hold it like that for a little while.

You should wait for a long time before you start doing sit-ups and for several months if you have had a cesarean section. Hard stomach exercises put a great strain on the stomach muscles and the bottom of the pelvis. It's better to lean your body back a little and sit with your legs pulled up. Then you will feel your stomach muscles contracting. Don't do anything that feels uncomfortable, especially if you have or have had pelvic problems. At the end of this chapter, you will find some simple, effective exercises to do at home if you have enough energy.

Otherwise, you might go for a long, brisk walk with the stroller to get exercise. Maybe you can meet up with a friend in the same situation. Now you need to become strong. You will need to maneuver the ever-growing baby and the stroller, and if you should make a trip to the store, there may be groceries to bring home. Avoid heavy lifting until the floor of your pelvis and any cesarean section scars have healed and any discomfort has disappeared. Get your whole body ready to lift: hold your stomach and lower abdomen taut and lift slowly and correctly. Bend your knees, stick your bottom out, and watch out for your back.

The Genital Area

Is your genital area starting to feel normal again? After four to six weeks, most of the stitches will have dissolved, and any tenderness around your scars will normally be gone. If you had painful stitches or tears, let them heal before you start your pelvic floor exercises seriously. Then you can—and should—begin.

A few women experience a kind of pressure in their vaginal area for a while after the birth—"as if it all were going to drop out." This normally disappears after a while. If it doesn't, go for a checkup. Is it difficult to control your perineal muscles? When you're urinating, see if you can stop the flow. If you can, you have good control. If you can't, put a finger in your vagina and squeeze. If you can feel your vagina is sort of gripping your finger; that's it. You will need to practice a lot. Squeeze together, pull up, and relax—again and again, in bed, in the kitchen, in the car, in front of the TV. Increase your efforts a little. Squeeze and pull up—higher—and higher—and higher. Hold for a bit. This also prevents urine leakage, a major problem for many women, especially as they age. Right now, though, it's probably more important that exercising your pelvic floor muscles helps your love life. Some women have actually told me that their sex life became better after their first baby, and they attribute this to these exercises, which make them much more aware of their vagina.

Sex

Some women find that the vaginal opening feels OK quite soon after birth, and they can't wait to resume their sex life. Nonetheless, it is sensible to wait until the bleeding has stopped and everything has dried up. Just as during menstruation, the womb is more susceptible to infection when the cervix is open to let fluids run out.

The most significant barrier to intercourse is often a lack of desire in the woman. Neither her body nor her hormones is ready for this. From nature's point of view, the purpose of intercourse is reproduction—neither needed nor desirable at the moment. The man essentially has just one form of biological behavior to promote reproduction: intercourse. Reproduction for a woman also includes giving birth and breastfeeding. From a biological point of view, although the man's body is ready to produce more children, the woman is still involved with producing the baby at hand. Women from other cultures tell of the rules for long sexual abstinence following a birth. Six months is normal.

The tiredness that results from having a baby is also an enemy to sexuality. Everyone knows this from past experience: "Not tonight, darling. I'm so tired." The man might help by taking over some of the work at night with the baby: changing, carrying, soothing. Two tired people go better together sexually than one who is tired and one who has had plenty of rest.

Some men also have problems with sex, and their desire seems to have disappeared. The birth may have been a difficult experience for the man. He may need some time to reconnect before he can associate the woman's body with sex again.

The most common situation, though, is that the woman is not interested yet, whereas the man wants the sex life to resume just as it was before. He may also have experienced a period of "sexual starvation" toward the end of the pregnancy.

Many women adapt to their partner's needs before they are really ready because they are so fond of their husband. They want to have warmth and tenderness and intimacy, and they know that men often connect this more closely with sex than do women. For women, desire lies as much in the head as in the body. Here humans are helped by their big brains once again. It is possible to decide to make conditions right for romantic feelings. Deliberately choose a day when you're not too tired, after a few months if not before. Make sure the baby is well fed. Dress up a little. Decide that you are going make yourself desirable to your partner, just as when you worked to get him to fall in love in earnest.

Often the woman, who probably wasn't so interested initially, makes an effort and suddenly finds that sex is wonderful—a bit strange at first, but it works. Both parties are excited. Did it feel different? From a purely technical point of view, it can. The vagina has been hugely stretched. But it is designed for this. It has folds, like a pleated skirt or an accordion. All the folds are stretched during the birth but go back together afterward. Even the opening to the birth canal is incredibly elastic. You might compare this to your lips, which can hold a pin but can also take a bite from a big apple. The muscles in the vagina can be exercised if they have become weak or if they were never particularly active before.

Some women suffer from vaginal dryness following childbirth. Using a neutral cream until your hormones make your vagina ready for sex is not an admission of failure. Many stores stock lubricant creams. Some women who suffer from soreness can benefit by using an estrogen pessary or cream a few times a week until they start to ovulate again. It's probably good for your sex life not to wait too long before you try having sex again. Many feel the time is right after the six-week checkup, if not before.

Breastfeeding as a Contraceptive

For many years, the old advice that breastfeeding prevented a new pregnancy was believed to be mostly superstition. This form of birth control was not recommended, at least in Norway, even though it was considered to have some effect on a worldwide basis. In more recent years, however, research has been carried out on the contraceptive effect of breastfeeding among well-nourished women from industrialized countries. Breastfeeding has been shown to be a very good contraceptive for the first six months after birth. Three main rules must be followed:

- The baby must be less than six months old.

- The baby must be exclusively breastfed, must not be given anything other than mother's milk, and must be breastfed at night.

- The mother must not have started menstruating again.

If you follow these rules, breastfeeding is just as safe as a minipill or an IUD (a copper coil): one to three women out of one hundred may become pregnant. This is a higher success rate than with a condom, for example.

Every time you breastfeed, you create hormones that prevent ovulation. You must do this at regular intervals throughout the day and night. If the gap between feedings is too long because the baby is starting to sleep six to eight hours per night, for example, ovulation will not be suppressed so effectively.

Since these new research results became known a few years ago, I have recommended breastfeeding as a contraceptive for many women for the first six months. So far, not one of them has become pregnant. Many really don't want to interfere too much with their body right after childbirth and think it's a good idea to have six months off before they choose another form of contraception.

Even after the first six months, breastfeeding is a reasonable contraceptive if you have not started your periods again. After one year, about 7 percent of women will become pregnant if they do not use an additional form of contraception. Combining breastfeeding and the use of a condom increases safety.

OTHER FORMS OF CONTRACEPTION

Many couples use condoms following a birth. It may seem fair for the man to take responsibility for contraception for a while as the women's body has been through so much. The condom also works as a prophylactic against infection for both partners.

If you want to use a contraceptive pill, a minipill is normally prescribed during the breastfeeding period (in contrast to standard contraceptive pills) because the minipill does not affect the amount of milk. One problem with the minipill is that you may experience light bleeding. A second disadvantage is that you must be careful to take the pill at around the same time every day to be as certain as possible not to become pregnant.

Ordinary combination contraceptive pills are the safest but normally are not recommended while breastfeeding. Both hormone coils and copper coils (IUDs) can be used, however. The hormone coil consists of tiny quantities of gestagen, the same ingredient in the minipill. This is very safe but may initially cause light bleeding and thereafter lighter periods or possibly no periods at all. It may be a good idea for you to wait about three months after the birth before a coil is inserted. This minimizes the risk of it falling out. One advantage of both the hormone coil and the copper coil is that they work just where they should and nowhere else. One of them can remain in your uterus for five years.

For some women, a contraceptive injection is an alternative. This also contains gestagen, which is injected every three months and forms a deposit. Light bleeding is common during the first few months, but such bleeding decreases among most women after a while, and between 20 and 50 percent of women stop menstruating completely. It can take time for menstruation to come back when you stop having contraceptive injections. They are fine for some people, especially for women who have problems remembering to use other forms of contraception. When you have this type of injection, its effects last for three months, so you can't just stop one day as you can stop other substances.

A little monitor is also available that shows "safe" days based on a test strip dipped in morning urine. Of every hundred women who use this system correctly, around six become pregnant in the course of a year. The advantage of this method is that you don't have to take pills, have a foreign body inserted, or use something in conjunction with intercourse.

THE ADVANTAGES OF BREASTFEEDING

In the old days, a woman was said to lose a tooth for every baby. This doesn't apply today; it had to do with poor dental care and diet, combined with a pregnant woman's tendency to snack all the time. Your bone structure will remain good and strong if you just make sure you take enough calcium to replace what you lose through your milk.

It's easy to note the positive effects that breastfeeding has on your body in the first few weeks after birth. Many women feel their womb contracting every time they breastfeed. The womb is an incredible organ. In the space of a short time, it will shrink to the size of a small pear behind the bladder, having stretched right up to the diaphragm before the baby was born. Much is made of the ability of the penis to almost double in size. But what about the womb, which can expand about fifty times? Of course, admittedly this expansion does take longer and happens rather less often.

In the long term, you will also benefit from breastfeeding. The Swedish professor Kerstin Uvnäs Moberg, who has done a lot of research into hormones, has demonstrated that the breastfeeding hormone oxytocin has a pacifying effect; reduces blood pressure, aggression, and anxiety; and strengthens the immune system. Women who breastfeed are less stressed and less often ill than women who do not breastfeed.

Most organs probably work best when they do what they are supposed to do. This also applies to the breasts. Breast cancer is the form of cancer that kills most women in the Western world today. This is particularly tragic when it affects younger women, who often have children to be looked after and should have lived for many, many years. A

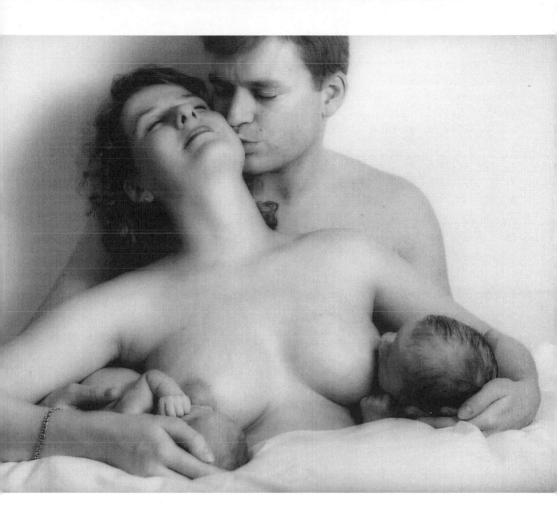

number of studies today show that breastfeeding reduces the risk of contracting breast cancer before menopause. A large, comprehensive study from Great Britain compared women who had developed breast cancer before they were thirty-six years old with similar, healthy women. Other known risk factors for breast cancer were taken into account, such as waiting a long time before the birth of the first baby, infertility, the use of contraceptive pills, the use of alcohol, inherited disposition to breast cancer, and so on. Breastfeeding nonetheless significantly reduces the risk. In general, it seems, the more children you have breastfed and the longer you have breastfed them, the better you are protected against contracting breast cancer before menopause.

Breastfeeding also appears to reduce the risk of ovarian cancer to some extent. This is a treacherous form of cancer, rarely discovered in time to be cured.

To strengthen and protect the pelvic floor:

- Press your legs together before you cough, sneeze, or lift something.

- See if you can stop the stream of urine when you urinate.

- Contract your pelvic muscles tightly, hold, and then relax; repeat 10 consecutive times, 5 times a day.

- Try to pull your pelvic floor up—up—up. Hold it there—and relax. Repeat 10 consecutive times, 5 times a day.

To start your stomach exercises:

- Pull your stomach in and hold it taut for a while.

- Lift your head when you lie on your back and look at your toes.

Extend this after a time, and:

- Sit with your legs pulled up. Lean back a little.

- Lie on your back. Raise your head and shoulders.

- Lift your shoulder toward the opposite knee. Swap over.

- Press your back against the floor.

For breastfeeding to work as a contraceptive:

- The baby must be less than six months old.

- The baby must be exclusively breastfed.

- Mother's milk only!

- The baby must be fed at night.

- You must not have started your periods again.

CHAPTER 21

. . .

What Passes into the Milk?

Many years as a doctor have taught me that some questions about breast milk come up over and over again when women come for postnatal checkups. The same problems come in by telephone, by mail, and through the media. Perhaps you are also wondering about these issues. Here are the answers to some of the most common questions:

Will it be all right for the baby if I eat normally while I am breastfeeding?
Yes. We don't discourage any types of food while you are breastfeeding these days, even though it is known from experience that some babies can react to what the mother eats.

I have heard that you should not eat cabbage, grapes, onions, or strawberries.
Some babies become unsettled when you eat these types of food. It's impossible to say in advance which baby will react to what, however. Try these different types of food carefully, and avoid them later if you notice that your baby reacts to them.

Is it true that I shouldn't eat fish, nuts, or oranges if I don't want my baby to develop an allergy to them?
No. We rarely give such advice to a breastfeeding mother, unless other family members have strong allergies to these things, as is occasionally true.

Some people say I should avoid dairy products if my baby has colic.
This seems to work for some mothers. Cut out all dairy products for a week and see if it helps. Then try drinking milk again. If your baby

becomes worse and then better again when you cut out the milk, continue to avoid dairy products.

But I thought I must drink milk when I am breastfeeding.
No. Eat carefully, and make sure you get plenty of calcium or calcium-rich foods, such as dark green vegetables like broccoli, parsley, spinach, and green cabbage; also eat sardines, crab, shrimps, figs, raisins, and almonds. You have lots to choose from. Sesame seeds contain large quantities of calcium and can be mixed into dough, porridge, or cereal mixes. You can also take calcium tablets.

I often drink gallons of coffee and cola during the course of the day. Does this have any effect?
If you have a very wide-awake, active, perhaps irritable baby who seldom sleeps for a long time, caffeine may be having an effect. Little of this passes into the milk, but caffeine corresponding to six to eight cups of coffee per day will have a tendency to accumulate in the baby. Try other soft drinks and decaffeinated coffee for a week and see if it helps.

Are tea and herbal teas OK when breastfeeding?
Yes. On the whole, tea is a good drink for breastfeeding mothers. Don't let it stand for too long, because the content of highly active substances, such as tannin, increases then. This works like caffeine. Green tea from China or Japan tastes good and is healthy. Herbal teas made with rosehips, chamomile, and peppermint are not dangerous. Rosehips also contain lots of vitamin C.

Can herbal teas have dangerous side effects?
Yes. Even medicinal herbs and so-called natural products are not to be toyed with. Use recognized brands that do not contain too many different ingredients. The great majority will be safe and healthy. It's difficult to know what you're getting when a number of herbs are mixed together. Anything that is claimed to have a medicinal effect may also have side effects. Women who have drunk large amounts of tea made from certain mixes of herbs have been known to experience vomiting, dizziness, sleeplessness, bleeding, and liver damage. Licorice root is found in some types of "breastfeeding tea." If the mother drinks gallons of this, the baby may suffer from lethargy, a weak cry, and weight loss; the mother may be become sleepy.

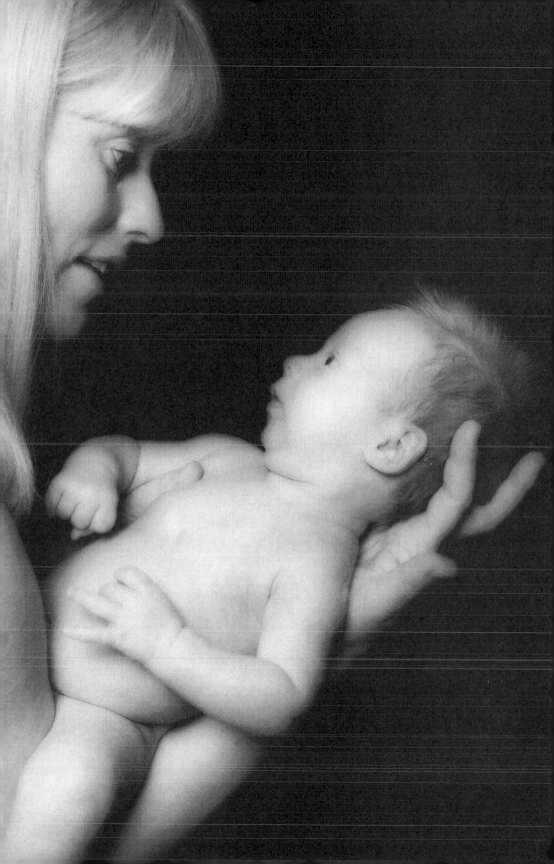

Will I produce more milk if I have a cup of "breastfeeding tea" from a health-food store?
Breastfeeding tea has not been proven in controlled tests to have any effects. The most important thing is to get into the habit of drinking tea before you breastfeed—mainly because fixed routines can help the letdown reflex. Farmers say that some cows begin to leak milk as soon as they come into the milking stall in the morning or when the farmer puts on some music.

Alcohol
Is it true that I can produce more milk if I drink beer?
Yes. A recent study indicates that this old advice might have something to it. To be on the safe side, you should drink alcohol-free beer. Alcohol-free malt beer also contains a lot of nutritional value and is an old, traditional breastfeeding drink.

I have heard that a glass of wine is good before breastfeeding.
We used to believe this. Now we know that as much as a whole glass of wine or a beer can hinder the letdown reflex, making it more difficult to get the milk out. A few cases have been described where large amounts of alcohol have destroyed this reflex for good.

Maybe I could have half a glass before most breastfeedings?
No. This would be too much in the course of the day, both for you and for the baby. Many breastfeeding women say that they very much enjoy a little wine or beer perhaps in the evening, however, when they are tired and have less milk. Then they relax and feel that the milk flows better.

Does that mean that the alcohol passes into the milk?
Yes. You will have at least the same amount of alcohol in your milk as in your blood. This means that there is a little alcohol in your breast-milk after a glass or two. Because the baby ingests this as food, it is nevertheless quite different than during pregnancy, when the baby's blood has the same alcohol content as the mother's blood and the baby is very vulnerable.

How does milk that contains alcohol affect the baby?

After a real binge, when the mother has a high level of alcohol, the breastfed baby can suffer alcohol poisoning, become listless, and suffer for several days, because the newborn cannot break down the alcohol in the way that we adults can. Tests have shown that babies also react to milk containing a low amount of alcohol. They drink a little less and sleep less well afterward—the opposite of what we used to believe.

Does anybody know what type of damage the baby can suffer and how much alcohol it takes to do this?

It appears that breastfeeding mothers who have a few alcoholic beverages every day can cause problems for their baby. These problems could include slow motor-skill development, a late start to crawling, and so on.

Is there any alcohol I can drink while I am breastfeeding?

Yes. There's no reason to believe that a single glass of wine, a beer, or a drink now and then will have any effect. Milk with a tiny percentage of alcohol still adds up to very little alcohol in the baby's system. The question is in quantity: a whole glass of wine, a strong drink, or half a bottle of beer gives an alcohol percentage of around 0.3 to 0.4 per thousand in the milk after half an hour to an hour. This breaks down by about 0.15 per thousand per hour. If you wait two to three hours before breastfeeding, this one glass will virtually be out of your system.

Do I have to be this careful all the time when I breastfeed? If so, I am going to give up soon!

No. When the baby is more than six months old and is starting to eat other types of food, you can miss a breastfeeding from time to time. This is a way to cope if you are longing to go to a party and drink socially: breastfeed your baby just before the party. Eat and drink what you want and then wait until the alcohol is out of your system before breastfeeding the next day. It will then be out of your milk as well. You could have problems with the expulsion reflex afterward, but this is rare.

I guess I should use a breast pump before I breastfeed after drinking alcohol?

Only if your breasts become uncomfortably full before enough time has gone by for you to breastfeed again. You don't need to do this for the sake of the milk. It will be free of alcohol at the same time as your blood is. The milk is not a finished product with a set composition once it is produced. The exchange between your milk and your blood is continuous.

Smoking

Is it really so dangerous to start smoking again after nine months of pregnancy and my baby has been born?
See if you can avoid starting again. Smoking while you breastfeed can create poorer milk quality and a smaller quantity of milk.

Why is there less milk when I smoke?
One reason may be that smokers often produce a little less prolactin, the hormone that controls the amount of milk. In addition, smoking has other effects on your body that are not good for the amount of milk. Furthermore, some smokers appear to spend less time breastfeeding their babies, so milk production is not adequately stimulated.

Why is the milk not so good if I smoke?
Many of the more than 4,000 substances in cigarettes—such as carbon monoxide, hydrocyanic acid, and tar—go into the milk. Nicotine has been studied the most. Nicotine gets into the milk particularly easily; concentrations in the breast milk are even higher than in the mother's blood.

How will this affect my baby?
Children of women who smoke are more likely to develop colic. They tend to cry more, are restless, and don't put on weight as much as children of women who do not smoke.

Since I do smoke, is it better if I don't breastfeed my baby at all?
No. From what we know today, experts think that mother's milk is so valuable for a baby that you should continue to breastfeed even if you can't quit smoking completely.

I have almost managed to stop smoking, but I can't give up cigarettes completely. When is my smoking least harmful for the baby?

The concentration of nicotine is at its highest in the milk just after you have smoked. So you should breastfeed first and then have a cigarette— or better yet, have half a cigarette, if you can't help it, and then don't smoke anymore before you breastfeed the baby again.

Can I use nicotine chewing gum while I breastfeed?

Yes, you can. Because you'll still get the nicotine in your milk, nicotine gum is not normally recommended for women who are breastfeeding. Nonetheless, it is better than smoking, because you avoid all the other substances in cigarette smoke. The level of nicotine will normally be lower after using nicotine preparations, such as chewing gum or patches, than after smoking a cigarette.

Apart from affecting my milk, does our smoking harm the baby in any way?

Yes. Babies who breathe in other people's smoke are ill more often. They are more likely to have lung infections, bronchitis, and earaches, for example, and may have a greater risk of developing asthma and generally of being admitted to the hospital. Smoking in the home also increases the risk of crib death. After the children of smokers become a bit older, they are more often absent from nursery and school because of illness.

Medicines

Do medicines pass into the mother's milk?

Most medicines you take will get into your milk to some extent. Ideally, you should use only medicines that you really need while you are breastfeeding.

Will my baby get a lot of my medicine?

Generally, the baby will get a very small dose. Some medicines are found only to a tiny extent in the breast milk; others are found in bigger quantities. You can breastfeed while taking most medicines, with a few exceptions. In general, tranquilizers or sleeping tablets taken over a long period of time may affect the baby. Certain hormones are not good, either. The conclusion in most books about this, nonetheless, is that it is normally better to breastfeed your baby even if you need medicinal treatment.

What about the contraceptive pill? Can I use that?
Normal combination pills can reduce the quantity of milk somewhat. As far as we know, the hormones in contraceptive pills do not affect breastfed babies.

Should I definitely avoid using any medicines in particular while I am breastfeeding?
Some cancer treatments and substances that depress the immune system should not be used when breastfeeding. Lithium, used for treating bipolar disorder, is not recommended at all. Certain strong antibiotics used to treat rare illnesses should not be combined with breastfeeding. The same applies to some heart medicines, which usually can be swapped for other medicine. Radioactive iodine and other seldom-used substances are also not recommended.

Ask your doctor or health adviser to check your medicine.

Environmental Toxins
There was something in the newspapers about dioxins and radioactivity in mother's milk. Is this dangerous?
Such substances can be found in the breast milk particularly of mothers who live in areas exposed to these substances. The same substances are found in dairy milk and in local water supplies, which are used for mixing milk substitutes, so avoiding them is not easy. Fortunately, the quantities are normally minute, with no harmful effects.

Environmental toxins such as PCB and pesticides are said to be found in greater quantities in breast milk than in cow's milk. Is this true?
Yes. This can happen. This is because human beings eat meat and fish and are thus higher up on the food chain than animals that just eat grass. Some environmental toxins are stored in the fatty tissues, and most of us go around with an odd layer or two. This is why active dieting is not recommended during the breastfeeding period; during periods of dieting, substances from "old" fatty tissues are used to create milk. Nevertheless, all studies show that in spite of this, breastfed babies turn out

healthier. The baby receives the greatest amounts of environmental toxins from the mother during pregnancy.

Can I do anything myself to prevent my baby from absorbing environmental toxins?

Yes. You can eat carefully. Eat good food, with plenty of vegetables. During the course of your pregnancy, you yourself built the whole of your baby's little body, and you also put some extra pounds on your hips and thighs. This is designed to be a nutritional reserve for use during breastfeeding. After you have been breastfeeding for a few months, the baby's milk requirement is fairly large. Most mothers start to lose their layer of fat from the pregnancy then and start to lose weight without trying to do so. If as much of your fat as possible is made of good, healthy food, with only a small quantity of animal products, the milk you create will also contain as few toxins as possible. If you continue being careful about what you eat, you will give your baby the best milk possible.

In conclusion, most of what you ingest will also reach your baby, first through the placenta and then through your breast milk. This does not mean that you need to live like a nun. Be particularly careful with medicines, smoking, and alcohol, and eat healthily—in other words, follow the rules that we would all do well to follow. For many people, having a baby is an incentive to follow such rules anyway. This is sensible because the baby is then likely to have healthy parents for many, many years to come.

Chapter 22

Reducing the Risk of Sudden Infant Death Syndrome

As a brand-new doctor, I was on call: At six o'clock on a winter morning, there came a desperate telephone call I will never forget: "Help! He's completely still. I don't think he's breathing!" A few minutes later, there was a screech of brakes. The young parents had driven to the hospital themselves because that was faster than waiting for an ambulance. On the way, the mother had tried to breathe life into her three-month-old baby; she had hit him in the chest and shaken him. It was no use. When we ran to meet them outside the hospital and I took the little body in my arms, the baby was still warm but completely limp, pale, and lifeless. No resuscitation techniques were of any use.

It was Sunday. The nineteen-year-old mother had had a visit from the baby's father, who lived in another city. Friends had been to visit; they had had a nice time that Saturday evening. The parents were proud when they showed off the baby, even though he was a bit miserable and had a stuffed-up nose. After he had drunk a whole bottle of milk, he was burped so that he would not suffer from colic as usual. His mother carefully aired the little one-room flat before they went to bed. She checked on the baby, who was sleeping, making tiny noises and small smiles in his sleep. Despite having had only a few hours' sleep, she woke early in the morning, at the time when the baby normally started crying, and worried when she didn't hear a sound. There he lay, the blanket partly over his head, completely still.

The parents were in shock. The mother screamed and cried, almost howling, and threw herself over the baby. The father stared at us in despair, completely gray. Comfort was meaningless. The little boy had been born a month early, a bit small and thin, but had come through with flying colors, was developing well and putting on weight, wriggling and babbling and beaming at everybody who talked to him.

The first time you experience something as serious as this, it sticks in your memory. But I have often thought about this particular sad story for another reason: it contains many of the factors known to increase the risk of sudden infant death syndrome (SIDS), also known as crib death.

Sudden and unexpected death among babies without clear cause used to be most common at around three months. Today this pattern seems to be changing. SIDS seldom occurs during the first month or after six months. Even with modern knowledge, we are often left without an answer why a particular baby has died. Perhaps the baby had a congenital weakness, which combined with other factors to cause death. Babies are particularly vulnerable between the ages of two and four months. During this time, major changes normally develop in their ability to regulate the activities of the heart and breathing.

SOME RECURRING CHARACTERISTICS

Nonetheless, some characteristics occur again and again in crib deaths. Although there are many exceptions, SIDS babies are typically found lifeless in the morning, in the winter, during the weekend. Typically they were a bit off color earlier, often with a virus infection. These babies often are lying on their tummy, perhaps with a blanket or comforter over the head, and are warmly dressed. Often the head is covered with a little cap, even indoors. A SIDS baby may have been born prematurely and/or been underweight at birth. In relation to the average mother, the mother of a SIDS baby is often young, single, and a smoker; has breastfed only for short periods; and has other children.

Tragically, one vital contributory cause of crib death over many years was the habit of putting newborn babies to sleep on their stomachs. A campaign began in the 1990s to put babies to sleep on their sides or, ideally, on their backs. After we began to put infants to bed on their backs again, the number of crib deaths are down to about one-fourth of what they used to be.

Some of this decrease is also because the rate of smoking among pregnant women went down considerably during the same period. Next to the baby's sleeping on the stomach, the mother's tobacco smoking is the greatest known risk factor for crib death. Smoking during pregnancy and tobacco smoke in a baby's surroundings are dangerous. Many studies show a two- to sixfold increased risk of SIDS among the children of parents who smoke. Families that have previously lost a baby in a crib death have a slightly increased risk of recurrence. Whether environmental factors or genetic problems cause this—or perhaps an interplay between the two—is uncertain. Babies who do not get breast milk also have a slightly higher risk. The same applies to twins.

Sleeping in the Same Bed—or Not?

More recently, terrified parents have called me: "Is it true that we shouldn't sleep in the same bed as the baby?" Experts have issued this advice because studies have shown that crib deaths occur more often when a baby sleeps in the same bed as the parents. What is not made clear is that this largely appears to apply to the babies of smokers. The alarm was raised when babies of African American women in the United States and Maori women in New Zealand were shown to be at increased risk for crib death. These people traditionally slept with their babies, a fact that was originally thought to be the reason for the higher risk. It was then shown that these same groups were underprivileged, smoked much more, and had a much poorer lifestyle than the groups with which they were being compared.

In countries where the mother normally has her baby close to her body day and night, crib death occurrence is extremely seldom. In industrialized societies such as the United States, the norm has long been for newborn babies to sleep alone. In such countries, many of those who deviate from the accepted norms and sleep with their baby likely do so because of poverty; dullness due to alcohol abuse, drugs, or medicines; lack of care; and so on. Such factors appear to varying degrees in the research reports.

Studies from cultures where the mother shares her bed with the baby but virtually never smokes indicated a low occurrence of crib death. This applies, for example, to the Japanese, Hong Kong Chinese, Bangladeshi, and South Sea islanders. A joint study of crib deaths in Norway, Sweden, and Denmark, conducted by the Medical Register of Births, showed that sleeping with the baby increased the risk of crib death only when the mother was a smoker.

One theory is that a smoker's breath contains too much carbon monoxide and other poisonous substances, which can weaken the baby's breathing center in the brain. Women who smoke while they are pregnant seldom give up smoking after the birth. It can therefore be difficult to make distinctions, but there seems to be an independent risk to smoking in pregnancy, even if the baby is not exposed to passive smoking after birth or to sleeping together with a mother who smokes.

If sleeping together with an infant proves to increase risk among groups other than smokers, we need to know it—but currently the research is not clear. The possible advantages of sleeping together must also be taken into consideration. Breastfeeding is benefited when the mother and baby sleep together, for example. Breast milk itself reduces the risk of crib death somewhat because breastfed babies are somewhat less liable to contract viral infections. Breast milk also appears to have a positive effect on the development of the brain, where the center for breathing is situated.

Professor James McKenna, who has done numerous studies in sleep laboratories, maintains that the phenomenon of newborn babies sleeping alone is relatively new. For the best possible type of sleeping, waking, and breathing patterns, McKenna claims, the baby needs the mother's body, or someone else's body, close by. "Babies need to be sloshed around," he says. He also says, "There is no such thing as a baby—there is always a baby and somebody." Young babies need to be stimulated and should always have somebody nearby.

Professor McKenna has carried out tests in the sleep laboratory using continual video filming throughout the night, with monitoring cables fastened to both the mother and the baby. He is not a specialist in crib death. The studies apply to healthy babies but are interesting in the context of SIDS as well. McKenna's conclusion is that a mother's proximity stimulates a sleeping baby through sounds, smell, touch, and movements. Lying on the stomach hardly occurs when babies sleep with their parents: the baby usually lies turned in toward the mother. The baby who sleeps with parents also spends fewer hours in the very deep type of sleep, from which it is difficult to wake—and suckles more often. Even so, mothers who sleep with their babies tend to get more sleep, because they don't have to spend time soothing their baby back to sleep in their own bed after breastfeeding and because the baby eventually manages to take the breast virtually without waking the mother.

This is thought-provoking. We know that crib death babies have stopped breathing for one reason or another. All babies have pauses in breathing, when their parents themselves hold their breath and wait. This is normal. These breathing pauses eventually stop by themselves. A baby prodded during such a breathing pause, however, will immediately start breathing again.

Babies must not become overheated. This could easily happen if the baby is lying in a narrow gap between the parents or if the mattress is very soft and warm, as with a water bed; if the comforter is big and heavy; or if the baby slides down under the covers. Think about this if you want to have your baby in your bed. This is particularly important if the baby is ill.

We must consider all the information available before recommending against mothers sleeping with their babies in general; babies still do this in most of the world and have always done so. Let us not forget all the experts' advice concerning newborn babies that in later years has proved not to be tenable. Here are a few examples: "You mustn't pick the baby up when she's screaming; don't feed him more than every fourth hour; don't let her suck from the mother's breast in the first twenty-four hours after birth; don't give more than one breast; don't let the baby sleep in the same room as the parents; don't let the baby sleep on his back." All of this advice has now been abandoned.

To reduce the risk of crib death:

- Let your baby sleep on his or her back.

- Do not smoke.

- Make sure the sleeping environment is not too hot.

- Give your baby breast milk.

- Let your baby sleep in the same room with you, within hearing distance.

- Do not share a bed with your baby if you smoke
  — or use tranquilizers
  — or have a water bed or a very soft bed
  — or if you are ill or very overweight.

RESUSCITATION

If you find your baby lifeless but warm, start resuscitation immediately:

- Dial 911; say that your baby is lifeless, and give your address clearly.

- Use your finger to clean out your baby's mouth of vomit or anything else.

- Lay your baby on his or her back on a hard floor.

- Gently thump the baby's chest.

To give mouth-to-mouth resuscitation:

- Carefully lift up the baby's chin a little.

- Place your mouth over the baby's mouth and nose and blow carefully five times. Note: The nose is the most important; you may just breathe into the nose if possible, without pressing the tip of the nose inward. Remember that the lungs are small, so use short breaths, and check that the chest is lifting a little.

- Often the baby will start breathing again. If not, and if you can't feel a pulse, use cardiopulmonary resuscitation (CPR), described below as well.

To give heart massage:

- Put two fingertips in the middle of the chest, just below the nipples. Press down 0.5 inch, five times, while counting out loud: 1 and 2 and 3 and 4 and 5.

To combine mouth-to-mouth resuscitation and heart massage (CPR):

- Blow once.

- Press on the chest five times at the rate of about one hundred times per minute. Continue to alternate between mouth-to-mouth and pressing on the chest until help arrives.

Ideally, more than one person should help: one should call for help, another should carry out artificial respiration and CPR. In reality, you are often desperately alone and must do the best you can. Blow carefully a few times and then shout for help while you give CPR; then blow again. Practicing on a large doll can be useful. If the very worst should happen, it might be a small comfort knowing that you at least tried to resuscitate the baby.

CHAPTER 23

Illnesses and Problems During the First Six Months

Let's turn our attention to a number of common illnesses and problems that your child may experience during the first six months. We will also look at some rare illnesses that you should know about. Discussed here are:

Bronchitis and inflammation
    of the lungs
Diarrhea and vomiting
Eczema
False croup and breathing
    problems
High temperature
Flat skull
Foreskin problems
Colds
Foreign body in the throat
Jaundice
Meningitis
Infection

Poor indoor climate
Insect bites
Stomachache
Umbilical hernia
Injury
Sunburn
Fungal infection
Projectile vomiting
Teething
Urinary tract infection
Rash
Hydrocele
Ear infection

BRONCHITIS AND INFLAMMATION OF THE LUNGS

Bronchial infections can spread to the lower bronchioles and may make the baby cough or breathe heavily. The respiratory syncytial virus (RS virus) and many other microorganisms may be the cause. Breathing becomes shallow and fast, the nostrils splay out when the baby breathes in, and the baby groans a little when breathing out. The baby looks pale and is generally run down, with a fever. Call the doctor. Holding the baby upright may help.

Diarrhea and Vomiting

Diarrhea and vomiting as a result of infection are rare among babies under half a year old, especially if they are breastfed. However, these conditions can be serious if they do strike because small babies become dehydrated relatively quickly. It is vital that the baby be given fluids. Breast milk is ideal and is tolerated better than anything else. A baby who will not eat or drink anything can often be comforted if she is offered the breast. Over the course of a few days, milk production will increase. If you are traveling in warm countries, it is sensible to continue to breastfeed your baby. This means that you must maintain your own level of fluids. If you are not breastfeeding your baby, try giving her a watery juice or a preparation from the drugstore designed to rehydrate the baby, both of which are tolerated better than cow's milk. If the baby becomes listless and will not take any fluids, see a doctor.

Eczema

Seborrheic eczema with "scales" is common in the first six months, and treatment by swabbing and washing is part of the baby's bathing and cleaning routine. Atopic eczema normally develops after the third month. It often manifests itself in small babies as patches of itchy, red, irritated, nubbly skin on the cheeks, around the mouth, and on the forehead, scalp, and neck. If the baby has this type of eczema and the family has a history of allergies, it may be sensible to avoid cow's milk, eggs, fish, and anything else to which any member of the family is allergic. This applies both during breastfeeding and when the baby moves on to solids. It is important not to irritate the skin. Avoid using soap on the baby and fabric softener in the washing machine. Soft cotton clothing is best. Wool and synthetics can irritate. Do not bathe the baby frequently, and use oil in the water. Avoid bubble baths. Steep a cotton bag containing bran in water for twenty minutes and then put the contents into the baby's bath. This will soothe the itching. Otherwise, you can obtain a number of creams and ointments—talk to your doctor.

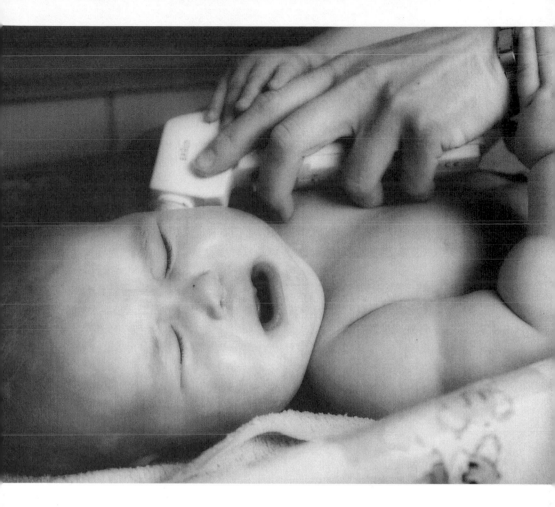

FALSE CROUP AND BREATHING PROBLEMS

Because the throat is so small in a newborn, even a small swelling can lead to breathing problems. This can occur in babies under six months but is more common between the ages of one and two years. If the baby develops a hoarse, dry cough, looks pale, or has problems with breathing, contact a doctor. If you know what this is because of previous episodes and the symptoms are not too serious, or while you are waiting for a doctor, you can hold the baby upright and allow the breathing of fresh cold air to help the baby breathe better. Stand in front of an open window or go outside with the baby. Let the baby sleep with the upper body raised a little and with the window slightly ajar.

HIGH TEMPERATURE

Fevers often occur in small babies, mostly caused by one of many infections they are likely to contract. A fever for a small baby does not necessarily indicate a serious illness. Young babies can be seriously ill without a fever, however. An increase in temperature is not always a bad thing. Viruses and bacteria are better fought with a moderate fever. Even with high fevers, seizures are rare in the first six months. You can help to reduce a fever by dressing the baby in light cotton clothing, letting the baby sleep in an airy room not warmer than 65°F, and perhaps washing the baby in lukewarm water and allowing the water to dry on the body and thus absorb some of the heat. Small newborn babies should be treated by a doctor if their fever does not have an obvious cause, such as when another family member is ill.

If medicines are used to bring down a fever, be careful to use the correct dose based on the baby's weight. Only use medicines designed for babies. Suppositories are often easiest to use because the risk of spillage is reduced and the baby is not forced to swallow something unwanted. Check on a sick baby during the night, setting an alarm clock if necessary. The baby's general appearance is as important as the temperature. Take action if the baby becomes listless and lethargic and will not eat.

FLAT SKULL

The skulls of small babies are soft and flexible. Some babies, after always lying on their backs, may end up with a flat or slanting skull. This normally corrects itself in time. It is important to ensure that even the baby who sleeps on the back should lie on the stomach or side when awake. Remember: "back to sleep, prone to play." Also, it is always a good idea to carry your baby because then there is little pressure on the head. Another good idea is to lie the baby with the head at the bottom of the bed on alternate occasions because the baby will turn the head toward the light after waking up.

FORESKIN PROBLEMS

The foreskin might seem a bit tight for baby boys who have not been circumcised. Pulling it back over the penis head can be impossible.

Earlier, doctors recommended stretching it regularly, but this only makes it worse. Today we advise against this because doing so may cause tears in the foreskin and leave scars. Besides, little boys seem to take care of the problem themselves by and by. Consider circumcision if the foreskin is so tight that it looks like a small balloon when the boy pees or if there is an infection. People from many cultures, including many in the United States, routinely circumcise their boys for various reasons, but no health gain has ever been proved. On the contrary, circumcision can sometimes lead to complications.

COLDS

A stuffed-up nose often distresses a small baby because babies usually breathe through their nose. Nosedrops for children can be used, but only for babies if really necessary. Let the baby sleep with the head raised; raise the head of the bed/crib/carrier without using a pillow. You could put some books underneath one end of the crib, for example. Try letting the baby "stand" while feeding. If the mucus is thick or crusty, drip a few drops of physiological salt water into the baby's nose. Small syringes are available to suck out the mucus. Eskimo mothers are renowned for using their own mouths to do this. Some people recommend dropping a few drops of breast milk into the baby's nostrils to loosen the crusts. Try a few drops from a small spoon. Try one nostril first. It is possible that antibodies in the milk, which are particularly important for the mucous membranes, may have a beneficial effect.

FOREIGN BODY IN THE THROAT

If you are certain that something is stuck in your baby's throat and your baby is in pain, has breathing difficulties, or is losing consciousness, proceed as follows:

- Hang the baby over your arm, head down.

- Tap sharply five times between the shoulder blades.

- Turn the baby onto the back, still head down.

- Press five times using two fingers on the chest between the nipples.

- Open the baby's mouth and see if you can find anything; if so, take it out. If you can't find anything, repeat the first four steps.

- Watch the baby carefully and make sure the breathing is all right.

- If the baby is unconscious, call 911. See page 231 for details of mouth-to-mouth resuscitation.

JAUNDICE

Many newborn babies become slightly jaundiced for the first few days. This is particularly common among babies born prematurely. Jaundice is caused by the fetus's need for extra red blood cells to get enough oxygen. When the baby starts to breathe air after birth, the excess blood cells are broken down and release a yellow substance, called bilirubin. The more bilirubin circulating in the baby's blood, the yellower the baby becomes, reaching an apex around the third to fifth day. Sometimes so much bilirubin is present that it may affect the baby. As a result, very jaundiced babies receive light treatment. The bilirubin breaks down more quickly under strong lights. Babies are often sleepy and lethargic when bilirubin levels are higher than normal.

What can you do yourself? Make sure that your baby gets enough food. The bowel empties itself after a meal because a reflex makes a full stomach send a message to either the large bowel or colon that more room will be needed and that the bowel must be emptied. The same happens with small babies—and with every dirty diaper, a jaundiced baby excretes some of the bilirubin as well. If the baby does not empty the bowel, some of the bilirubin is reabsorbed and recirculates. Research has shown that a baby who is breastfed at least eight times per day is less susceptible to jaundice than a baby who is fed less often.

Getting a jaundiced, sleepy baby to suck can be difficult. Don't let the baby sleep for more than three hours at a time during the day. Wake him up well ahead of time; carry, rock, and swing the baby a little; undress him; massage the soles of the feet and the hands; and let the baby lie with knees bent up while feeding. Allow plenty of time; pauses are normal. If getting the baby to suck is impossible, express a little milk and put a few drops on the baby's lips for temptation. Stimulate your breast before you feed your baby so that the milk comes as soon as the baby starts to suck. If you do not have enough milk yet, give a supplement, but let the baby breastfeed first.

Another piece of advice may help a little. Light treatment was found to be effective when jaundiced babies placed close to the window recovered more quickly than those who lay further away from daylight. Babies who are slightly jaundiced but who are below the level for light treatment, then, may well benefit from daylight. Make sure the room is nice and warm, and let your baby, or part of your baby, lie naked near the window. Avoid direct sunlight.

Occasionally, blood type problems lead to baby jaundice. If the yellow color does not decrease in the course of the first two or three weeks, or if the jaundiced baby is lethargic and does not put on much weight, see a doctor. Jaundice that develops later or carries on for a long time must be treated by a pediatrician.

MENINGITIS

One of the most terrifying infections is infectious meningitis. In addition to a fever and general lack of well-being, bleeding can occur under the skin, which aids the diagnosis. Contact your doctor if you see warning signs, such as small spots of blood that do not go pale in the way that normal rashes do when you press on them using a glass. Larger, bluish bleeding under the skin is another warning sign. Children may have a stiff neck and cry when you lift their heads, with their chin toward their chest. You can sometimes feel that the fontanel, the soft point on top of the head, is taut. These serious symptoms of meningitis are rare, fortunately, but they can appear quickly and may be life threatening. When my own babies were ill with a high fever, these were the symptoms I looked for at regular intervals during the day and once or twice in the night. I would set an alarm clock and look under the baby's pajamas for skin changes.

INFECTION

The newborn baby already has a number of protective antibodies from the placenta. These break down to a large extent during the first six months. Breastfed babies also get large amounts of antibodies through their mother's milk and are less vulnerable to infection. Breastfeeding is no guarantee against infection, however: all babies can become ill. Try to avoid the risk of infection for small babies. Ask people with colds and other illnesses to keep their distance. A breastfeeding mother who develops a bronchial infection could use a mouth mask for the first days while at her most infectious; after a few days, the milk will contain antibodies to fight this infection. Siblings with colds should avoid kissing the baby on the mouth at this time. Cuddling a little foot, for example, will do just as well. Our youngest child maintained when she was small that her big toe was particularly long because her big brothers used to not only kiss it but suck it when they had colds and wanted to give her a cuddle.

POOR INDOOR CLIMATE

Air out the house frequently and avoid all indoor smoking when a new baby is present. Passive smoking increases the risk among babies of illnesses such as asthma, bronchitis, lung infections, and meningitis. Healthy babies should spend some time outside every day if the climate is suitable, as this strengthens the mucous membranes.

INSECT BITES

Wasp stings, one of the most common forms of insect bites, can be serious for a newborn baby. Be particularly vigilant if the baby is stung on the neck or face. If the baby becomes pale or has breathing difficulties, contact a doctor immediately. A local anesthetic ointment designed for this use can soothe the pain. The old wives' remedy of putting half a raw potato cut side down on the bite can also help as can other traditional remedies, such as cooling the bite with ice.

STOMACHACHE

Stomachache is often related to colic, which you can read about in chapter 18. Babies who will not eat or whose bowel movements change considerably, or who scream when you press on their stomach and pull their legs up, may be ill and should be checked by a doctor. A twisted bowel may be causing problems, for example. Blood may be seen in the bowel movement. Occasionally it may be seen coming from a visible tear in the anal opening. Report any other form of bleeding to your doctor.

Umbilical Hernia

A small bulge around the navel will most often retract during the course of the baby's first year. The swelling is usually related to a temporary weakness in the ring of muscles around the navel. The fetus needed a good opening there to accommodate the umbilical cord. Now the opening there just needs time to narrow. Umbilical hernias generally are not painful, and what you see when the baby is crying are not intestines bulging out.

Injury

Fortunately, injuries among small babies are rare. The most common injuries happen when babies fall from changing tables, sofas, or similar places. Head injuries are usually serious. Babies who hit their heads heavily should be kept under observation for the next eight to ten hours. They should be woken up from their sleep every other hour to make sure that they have not lost consciousness. If you cannot wake a baby whose head has just been hit, contact your doctor even if the baby is unconscious for only a few minutes. The same applies if the baby is pale and listless or starts vomiting.

Sunburn

On the whole, small babies should not be exposed to direct sunlight and should be kept mostly in shade. Dress the baby in cotton clothing that covers the limbs, rather than using sun lotion. Sunstroke occurs when the head has become too hot and the brain is irritated. The newborn baby is particularly vulnerable to this, with a large and often hairless head. Always make sure the baby wears a sun hat with a brim when out in the sun. If the head becomes too warm, cool it down a little. Soak the sun hat with water to produce a cooling effect.

Fungal Infection

Thrush, a fungal infection in the mouth, seldom worries the baby, although a sore in the mouth can occasionally develop, and the baby may refuse to suck. Thrush looks like a white, milky coating. Make sure you boil your baby's pacifier and bottle teats. Fungal medicines prescribed by a doctor will help. Put a compress on your index finger and dry out the baby's mouth before rubbing the solution into it. Try using a thin layer of material on your finger or a cotton swab for this. The baby can infect the breasts, causing the mother to become sore and to need treatment.

Projectile Vomiting

Most babies vomit from time to time with their vomit spurting from the mouth. This is normally of no significance. Real projectile vomiting usually becomes apparent when the baby is a few weeks old. It is slightly more common among boy babies and is due to a slight narrowing of the exit from the stomach. Often the baby vomits an hour or so after being fed. If this happens after most feedings, and if the baby is hungry and feeding well but is not putting on weight, have a specialist see the baby. A small operation may be needed on the pylorus muscle, which regulates the amount of flow from the stomach down to the bowel. Projectile vomiting should not be confused with normal gulping and minor vomiting.

Teething

The baby may appear miserable and uncomfortable, but teething itself does not cause a fever. The reason teeth often appear after the baby has had a fever is that the gums are more readily absorbed during a fever. The baby often appears to have tender gums. Something solid to bite on, such as a rubber ring, can help. Drugstores sell a soothing preparation to rub into the gums. This is not normally necessary, however.

Urinary Tract Infection

Diagnosing urinary tract infections in babies can be difficult. General lack of energy, poor appetite, and a slow increase in weight may all be symptoms. Many, but not all, babies run a fever. Special bags can be attached to the baby to take a urine sample.

Rash

Infectious childhood illnesses with rashes seldom occur in the first six months. Impetigo can occur at any age and is highly infectious. The head is usually affected first, but the small pustules can appear everywhere. When they burst, they form an open, red, weeping surface, which develops yellow scabs. Impetigo is a streptococcal infection. All pustules or sores need to be disinfected. The doctor can prescribe an ointment to deal with these bacteria.

Hydrocele

The scrotum in small baby boys can swell up without appearing to irritate the baby unduly. The body normally absorbs the extra fluid after a while. If the baby also has an inguinal hernia with the peritoneum or intestines bulging out in the crotch when it cries, an operation may be required.

Ear Infection

An earache, although common among small babies, can be difficult to detect. It is rarely seen in a breastfed baby. Typically, the baby wakes up screaming because of changes in the pressure in the ear just after beginning to suck or after being put down to sleep. If the baby cries inconsolably and twists the head, try pressing carefully with your fingers just in front of the ear. The baby will often react, indicating that this hurts. In this case, see a doctor. Having the baby lie with the head raised can help the earache. Carrying the baby with the head upright and encouraging feeding in a "standing" position can also help. Warmth, such as a warm hand over the ear, can soothe the pain a little. The baby should wear a hat to properly cover the ears.

CHAPTER 24

· · ·

From Now On, Everything Will Get Better and Better

Little Frances, whom I told you about at the beginning of this book, is now six months old, and we are still in touch. She gets sweeter and more amusing by the day. She stretches her arms out toward her parents and laughs in amazement whenever they do anything she thinks is amusing. She is sitting up, albeit very unsteadily, and joins in with everything that is going on. She can do things herself to get what she wants: put a crust of bread in her mouth, grab hold of a toy, chew it, throw it away. She can pull herself across the floor a bit and can grab something that was quite out of reach just one month ago. She thinks life is wonderful.

An Ever-Increasing Love

It is hardly pure chance that she starts to show love to those whom she knows at around the time she is starting to learn to be able to move away from them. When she was younger, as long as she lay in somebody's arms, she was safe. Now that she is increasingly able to move herself, something must make her want to stay close even when no one is actually watching over or holding her. The fact that she wants to be with those to whom she is closest is part of the safety network she is developing.

As Frances finds her own ways of creating contact, the family becomes more and more fond of her. She is exciting and amusing to be with, not just little and helpless. Her grandparents are besotted with her. Had Frances had siblings, this would have increased the opportunities for play and communication—and also for jealousy. Many children first really react negatively when a new baby starts to get himself

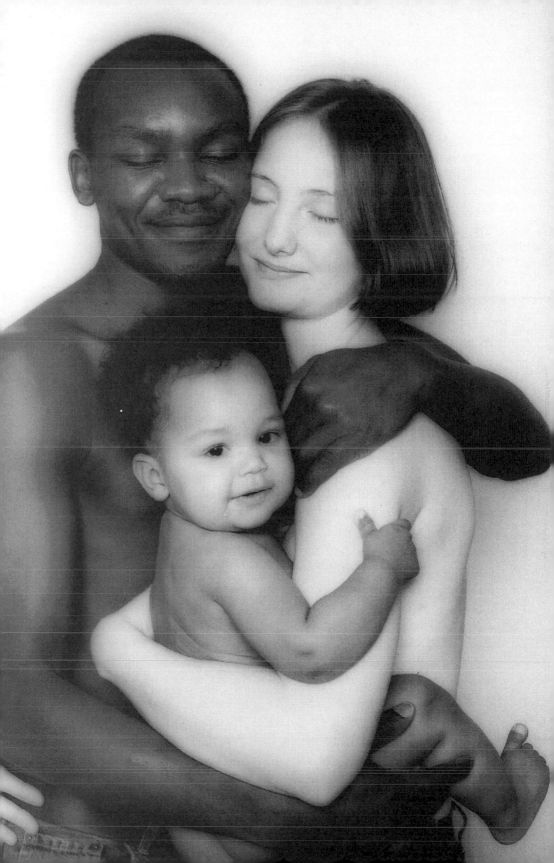

noticed and receives plenty of attention for new skills and abilities, for charm and funny behavior.

Increased Freedom

Frances's mother and father feel that having a baby has been tiring, even though everything has gone well for them, with no major initial problems. Frances has been healthy and has received plenty of breast milk. Ann, who used to wonder whether she really had enough milk to exlusively breastfeed her big daughter, has finally relaxed. Now her daughter is starting to have other types of food as well, although she is still breastfed at every meal—usually first, sometimes last, and occasionally, when necessary, right in the middle. Ann sometimes ends up with porridge half over her breasts, a real mess. It is fun to give Frances new types of food, new tastes, new textures. She spits in disgust or swallows enthusiastically, depending on what it is. She is easily distracted and must be diverted with a toy so she doesn't grab the spoon. She lets go of the breast and turns with interest as soon as her mother starts talking to someone else. Sometimes Ann has to feed her without anyone else in the room, even in the daytime.

Ann is looking forward to having a little more time to herself. Soon she will be able to go out for half a day without having to use the breast pump first because Frances can now drink juice. In two weeks, they are going to a thirtieth birthday party, and Ann is going to drink plenty of wine and then wait the next day before breastfeeding, when all the alcohol is out of her blood and her milk. At last Ann is beginning to feel that she has control over her own body again. The postnatal gymnastics and long walks with the stroller have helped. So has breastfeeding in the last few months. After four months of breastfeeding, the layers of fat began to slide off her stomach and thighs without her even trying. Her whole little family thinks her breasts are marvelous. She no longer wakes up with a full feeling in them, and leakage at the wrong moments has all but disappeared. Joe is very impressed with her soft, round breasts. He even admits to having tasted her milk—"like warm milk and honey."

More Energy

Their love life has really taken off again. Those "wobbling rolls of fat," as Ann called them, have gone. Joe's nearest and dearest looks like herself again. He thinks she has never looked so good as she does now. She feels a new intensity in their relationship, an awareness that their sex life is not just a game; it can actually lead to a whole new person, just like Frances. Ann's genitals are fine now. In fact, her pelvic floor exercises have given surprisingly pleasant results.

Of course, Ann is still a bit tired because Frances still needs feeding during the night, even though she has slept through sometimes. But it's not so awful to be woken up when you can get plenty of sleep at other times. It's no longer as strange and disturbing as it was in the beginning. It's almost easier to breastfeed at three o'clock in the morning and then go to sleep again than to be woken at five o'clock in the morning by a starving baby who wants to get up. The fog or fuzzy feeling of breastfeeding is over. A zest for life, for new experiences, and for getting together with friends has replaced her peaceful introspection.

Who Is Going to Take Maternity/Paternity Leave Now?

Plenty of leave is still owing. Joe wants to be at home with Frances for a good long while. He thinks it is time to change roles anyway, after half a year. He and Ann discussed with me how the leave would be split between them.

"I want to be the most important person in her life for a bit, too," Joe told me. "Anyway, I could do with some time at home enjoying life."

But Ann does not want him to take a large part of their leave: "I was the one who was pregnant, had morning sickness, got diarrhea from the iron pills, had to stay in bed because I was bleeding. I'm the one who made this baby from my own body, apart from one single cell you contributed at the start. I'm the one who risked my health and my pelvis and got stretch marks in order to have her. Even though it has been fun, it has also been very tough, and we didn't know how it would work out. I have struggled through the most tiring period. I am just beginning to feel my old self again, everything is going well, and she is wonderful. Can't you see that now comes the real reward?"

Joe looks a bit flat and admits that there have been major differences in the input so far. "But surely you want her to have a close relationship with her father as well? It isn't the same when you are always around."

And Ann retorts, "You already have plenty of time with her in the evenings and on the weekends, and she's just more and more taken with you. I think newborn babies need their mother most at the beginning. After all, there is a reason why it is the woman who carries the baby, pushes her out, and feeds her, all from her own body."

They carry on, the two of them arguing, and finally come to an agreement. One of Ann's friends couldn't wait to get back to work again. She started again after four months, while her husband looked after things at home and even took the baby to her at work once a day. Everyone is different. The mother must take maternity leave for the first six weeks after the birth.

More and more often I hear of women who feel pressured to go back to work before the end of their maternity leave, while the husband "skims the cream, just when it all starts being fun." Perhaps it is sensible to let the mother be the one who has the final word in these matters, at least for the first eight or nine months. It also makes it easier to continue breastfeeding. Of course, the husband must be involved, and so many exciting things are happening with new fathers who are 100 percent involved in looking after their new baby.

In previous generations, it was said that it takes one baby to make a mother, but three to make a father. These days, fathers tend to be involved in quite another way, right from the start, and today's young dads are often highly experienced after one baby. The father is invaluable for the family's well-being. Nonetheless, the woman is, without doubt, best equipped biologically—even beyond the obvious things like hormones and breasts—to take care of a baby at the beginning. Women are more sensitive to sound, smell, and touch than men. They find it easier to read their newborn baby's facial expressions, and they use gentler movements when they touch the baby. They also have a more calming effect with their soft, light, rhythmic voice patterns.

Recent research has indicated that women go through notable changes in personality during pregnancy. They become more peaceful, less anxious and aggressive, more aware of other people's feelings and of communication without words. This is not so surprising, perhaps, and very practical for giving a newborn baby the best possible care at the start.

Dad Becomes More and More Important

The father's significance increases week by week. Experts wonder whether the fact that he is a bit different has a special significance for the baby's development. This does not mean that men are unable to care for tiny babies, but simply that women generally, and not surprisingly, have an advantage in this respect. The changes that occur in women around this time have been called nature's christening gift for the newborn baby.

Many women find it difficult to hand their baby over, even to the father. At the beginning, this feeling of possessiveness can benefit the baby because he or she ensures constant attention from the mother. If both mother and father feel that the mother is the only one who can give this attention, though, it may create a vicious circle. Other people, and primarily the father, must eventually be allowed to take part, as this is best for everybody involved. Slightly older babies feel safe when they find out that several people will look after them and love them. An extended family acts as a safety net in many ways. Nonetheless, it is not good for a baby to be sent back and forth between parents who do not live together before the child reaches a certain maturity. This should not be done while the baby is still so small that it affects breastfeeding.

A woman's hormones and instincts help largely at the beginning. Research into animals shows that the young themselves quickly become the most important stimulus for care from their parents, independent of hormones and gender. Male birds are just as important as females. Among mammals, the mother necessarily plays a special role. If you remove all the care hormones from a female rat that has given birth, she still looks after her young. If you take away her young, however, this maternal behavior will soon stop. A chimpanzee will carry her dead baby around for a few days, but when the baby gives no response, the mother's interest wanes, and finally she puts it down.

THE LIMITS OF DEVOTION

Ann is partly looking forward to getting back to the adult world of working life, but she is dreading leaving Frances. She has seen friends struggle with bad consciences and families who needed complicated timetables to function each day. The feeling that one should give up everything else for the child sits there, gnawing away. But life consists of compromises, of course, and looking after your children, along with everything else you want to have in life, is just such a continual compromise. We have to live with this. Make sufficient time, even though it would be better for your baby to have yet more. But if your baby took up all of your time, there wouldn't be enough time left to make progress at work, be a good partner and provider, enjoy friends, and have other interests. As a result, we would probably be less satisfied, less happy, and consequently function less well as parents. Don't despair: just make sure that your first priority is to make sure that your baby is well looked after, even if you can't do it all yourself.

In an entertaining book called *Natural Parenting,* author Susan Allport includes a chapter called "The Limits of Devotion," in which she looks at the sometimes doubtful behavior of animals and human beings toward their young. Animals that have a short life span, such as rats and small birds, generally are good parents, steered largely by instinct. Larger animals, which live longer, are not automatically good parents. Some become confused and scared when they have their first litter and end up eating the babies. Animals often ignore the runts of the litter. Sometimes they leave their young alone and helpless, especially when food is in short supply. The time when the mother leaves her young or scares them away is also a compromise. Often the offspring would be better off staying with their mothers for longer. But the mother has to go on, put herself first, become fertile again, and have more young.

The better the care apes get from their mothers as babies, the better they function as parents. They have to learn the art of parenting. It is the same with people. In our part of the world, with small families, increasing isolation, and minimal experience of new babies among many people, this can be a major problem for first-time parents. Perhaps looking after children should be valued more highly than it is today. Perhaps parenting courses should become just as common as prenatal classes. After all, giving birth is something that the body does largely by itself. It is the next weeks, months, and years that are the greatest challenge.

People in Glass Houses . . .

One thing is sure. Many of us try giving advice, and yet we ourselves sit in glass houses and certainly haven't gotten it all right all the time. When I had my first baby at the age of twenty-three, I felt that I was reasonably well prepared. I had been intensely interested in babies for as long as I could remember and had looked after my little sister and other people's children. My baby was wanted, and I soon fell in love with the little soul. Nonetheless, the demands came as a shock. This screaming little person had the right to keep me up at night. I always had to be there to change him and feed him, no matter what I wanted to do. Caring for him was overwhelmingly exhausting and took over my whole day. I often felt badly treated and frustrated that this baby, to whom we devoted so much love, sometimes seemed so dissatisfied.

Then our second child arrived. Suddenly, changing the baby was a nice break, and breastfeeding was a positive rest compared to dealing with a toddler in the middle of the terrible twos. Our third child was pure pleasure, with older siblings and lots of people around to help. Very few women get this far in Norway these days. The average is around two children each. We never manage to become experts through our own experience. As a result, we need to learn from each other.

When Should We Have Another Baby?

Ann and Joe have used breastfeeding as a contraceptive up until now. They are wondering when is the best time to have a second baby. Not right away, anyway. Ann wants to use an IUD for at least a year. When does the body really get back to normal? When is there the least risk of sibling rivalry? Is it better to take two periods of maternity leave close together or to have a good gap in between, with regard to one's career?

One thing is certain: Ann and Joe are determined to plan well for the next baby. Eat well, take cod liver oil, keep away from smoke and pollution. Ann is already taking vitamins and folic acid. She says she is much more aware now than she was before she had Frances. Then they thought nothing could go wrong. Now they have experienced much more. They have managed to survive the life crisis that can occur in having a first baby. Granny shakes her head warningly when they talk about having another baby and reminds them that "one is one and two are ten," but they are quite sure that if everything goes all right with the next pregnancy, it will all be a lot easier with the second baby.

Before a planned pregnancy, it is sensible to:

- Eat carefully.

- Take folic acid and other vitamins.

- Stop smoking.

- Get physically fit.

- Avoid harmful substances.

Resources

Publications for Parents

Bestfeeding: Getting Breastfeeding Right for You by Mary Renfrew, Chloe Fisher, and Suzanne Arms (Berkeley, CA: Celestial Arts, 2000).

Birth Without Violence by Frederick Leboyer (New York: Knopf, 1975).

Birthing from Within: An Extra-Ordinary Guide to Childbirth Preparation by Pam England, C.N.M., M.A. and Rob Horowitz, Ph.D. (Albuquerque, NM: Partera Press, 1998).

Breastfeeding and Natural Child Spacing: The Ecology of Natural Mothering by Sheila Kippley (New York: Penguin Books, 1978).

The Breastfeeding Answer Book by La Leche League International (Schaumborg, IL: 1997).

Breastfeeding Your Baby by Sheila Kitzinger (New York: Knopf, 1998).

Breasts, Bottles and Babies by Valerie A. Fildes (Edinburgh University Press, 1989).

Complete Book of Pregnancy and Childbirth revised and expanded edition, by Sheila Kitzinger (New York: Knopf, 1989).

The Descent of Woman by Elaine Morgan (Souvenir Publishers Ltd. 1985).

The Human Sexes: A Natural History of Man and Woman by Desmond Morris (New York: Dunne Books, 1998).

Mother Nature: Maternal Instincts and How They Shape the Human Species by Sarah Blaffer Hrdy (New York: Ballantine Books. 2000).

A Natural History of Parenting by Susan Allport (Three Rivers Press, 1998).

The Nursing Mother's Companion by Kathleen Huggins (National Book Network, 1999).

The Womanly Art of Breastfeeding by Judy Torgus (Franklin Park, IL: La Leche League International 1997).

Your Amazing Newborn by Marshall H. Klaus, and Phyllis H. Klaus (Reading, MA: Perseus Books, 1998).

VIDEOS

Mark-It Television Associates, *Breastfeeding: Coping with the First Week.* www.Markittv.com PO Box 21207, Waco, TX 76702-1207
800-299-3366
or in the UK 7 Quarry Way, Stapleton, Bristol, BS16 1UP. England. Tel 0117 939 1117/8

Nylander, Gro. *Breast Is Best.* (34 minutes) Award-winning video available in 30 languages. For information on national distributors contact Health-Info, Video Vital, fax + 47 22 56 19 91, e-mail: health-info@videovital.no. A questionnaire for self-study of this video is available in several languages.

Car Seat Safety, Injoy Productions and Cosco Video, 1998 (15 minutes).

Helping a Mother to Breastfeed: No Finer Investment, The Royal College of Midwives. London: Healthcare Productions Ltd. 1990. Healthcare Productions Ltd., Unit 1.04, Bridge House, Three Mill Lane, London E3 3DU www.healthcareproductions.co.uk

PUBLICATIONS FOR PROFESSIONALS

Bedsharing Promotes Breastfeeding. J. McKenna, S. Mosko, C.A. Richard.. Pediatrics 100:214-9,1997.

Breastfeeding. A Guide for the Medical Profession. R.A. Lawrence. Mosby 1999.

Breastfeeding and Human Lactation. J. Riordan, K.G. Auerbach. (2nd ed.) Jones and Bartlett Publishers, Inc. 1999.

Breastfeeding and the Use of Human Milk. American Academy of Pediatrics. 1997;100:1035-39.

The Breastfeeding Atlas. Barbara Wilson-Clay and Kay Hoover. Austin, TX, LactNews Press, 1999.

Breastfeeding: How to Support Success. T. Vinther, E. Helsing. World Health Organization, Regional Office for Europe, Copenhagen, 1997.

Breastfeeding Matters. M. Minchin. Sidney Australia: Alma Publications 1985.

Evidence for the Ten Steps to Successful Breastfeeding. World Health Organization 1998. WHO/CHD/98.9.

HHS Blueprinting for Action on Breastfeeding. U.S. Department of Health and Human Services. Washington, DC: Department on Health and Human Services, Office on Women's Health, 2000.

How Breast Milk Protects Newborns. J. Newman. Scientific American. December 1995.

Is Breastfeeding Beneficial in the UK? Statement of the Standing Committee on Nutrition of the British Paediatric Association. Archives of Disease in Childhood 1994;71:376-380.

Maternal and Infant Assessment for Breastfeeding and Human Lactation. K. Cadwell, C. Turner-Maffei, B. O'Connor, A. Blair. Jones and Bartelett Publishers, Inc. 2002.

Medications and Mothers' Milk. T. Hale. Pharmasoft Medical Publishing 2001.

The Optimal Duration of Exclusive Breastfeeding. A Systematic Review. Michael S Kramer and Kahuma Ritsuko. World Health Organization. WHO/NHD/01.08 WHO/FCA/CAH/01.23.

Successful Breastfeeding.M Royal College of Midwives, London, UK. (3/e). Churchill Livingstone. Elsvier Sciences 2001.

Unsupplemented Breastfeeding in the Maternity Ward. Positive Long-term Affects. G. Nylander, R. Lindemann, E. Helsing, E. Bendvold. Acta Obstetrica et Gynecologica Scandinavica 70; 1991: 205-9.

A Warm Chain for Breastfeeding. The Lancet: Editorial. Vol. 344; 1994:1239-1240.

Index

father
  cesarean section and, 64
  crying infant and, 184
  importance of, vii–viii
  role at birth, 7–10
  role of, 3, 35–45, 249
  sex and, 211
fatty acids, 115–116
feeding, night, 107, 158–159, 199–200
fertility monitor, 214
fetal membrane, 80
fever, 236, 242
fluid, 82, 121, 234
food. *See also* breast milk; breastfeeding;
    diet
  bottle feeding, 172
  breast milk and, 217–220
  crying and, 194
  solids, 159–160
forceps delivery, 66
foremilk, 117–118, 187
foreskin, 106, 236–237
formula
  bottle feeding, 167–168
  cow's milk and, 162
  doubts about, 154
  fatty acids in, 115–116
  preparation of, 168–169, 172–173
  weight gain and, 122
fungal infection, 110, 241–242

genital area healing, 210
gripping reflex, 27, 64, 174–176
gut, 129

hair loss, 88
hand milking, 72–74, 158
head, 102, 176, 241
health adviser, 99–100
hearing, 3–4, 13, 70, 178–179
heart defect, 69
heart massage, 231
hemoglobin level, 17
hemorrhoids, 85–86, 90
hernia, inguinal, 243
hernia, umbilical, 241
home birth, 91–92
home, return to, 92–93
homing, 125–126
hormone coils, 213
hormones
  as aid, 5–6
  breastfeeding and, 6–7, 198
  hair loss and, 88

in mammals, 39
of newborn baby, 19
postpartum blues and, 56
relaxin, 87
hospital
  birth, institutionalized, 47–48
  breastfeeding support of, 33–34
  discharge from, x–xi
  help from, 100–101
hydrocele, 243

IgA (immunoglobin A), 124–127
immune system, 124–127, 134
immunoglobin A (IgA), 124–127
impetigo, 243
incubator, 71
infant development
  physical, 176–177, 182
  psychological, social, 179–181, 182
  of reflexes, 174–176, 181–182
  of senses, 177–179
infection
  avoiding, 239–240
  ear, 243
  fighters in breast milk, 127–128, 129
  mastitis, 137–139
  thrush (candida), 140, 153, 241–242
  urinary tract, 242
insect bite, 240
instincts
  maternal, 38–39, 249
  of mother and child, 5–6
  paternal, 7, 10
  procreation, 40–41
intelligence quotient (IQ), 115
intercourse, 210–212, 247
interferon, 128
intravenous feeding, 151
IQ (intelligence quotient), 115
iron, 81, 119, 128, 160
isolation of mother, 97, 98, vii
IUDs (copper coils), 212, 213
jaundice, 27, 238–239
jealousy, 42–43

kangaroo method, 73–74

Lactobacillus bifidus, 105, 118, 128
lactoferrin, 128
La Leche League, 100
latching on, 21–22, 25–26
letdown reflex, 28, 136, 151–152, 220
light treatment, 27, 238, 239
lithium, 224

location reflex, 174
loneliness, 184, 186
love, 244, 246
lungs, inflammation of, 233–234
lying in, 47–48, 93–94

macrophage, 127
massage, 27, 28, 192, 231
mastitis, 31, 137–139
maternal instincts, 38–39, 249
maternity/paternity leave, 247–248
maternity ward
  crying in, 193–194
  early discharge from, x–xi
  feeding in, 154, 156
  length of stay in, 92
  rooming with newborn, 198
meconium, 105, 117
medicine, 223–224, 236. See also breast milk
    as medicine
melatonin, 201
memory, 126, 127, 179
meningitis, 239
midwife, 54–55, 63
milk. See breast milk; cow's milk
milk ducts, plugged, 136
milk substitute. See formula
minerals, 119–120
minipill, 212, 213
motherhood, 51, 96–97
mouth-to-mouth resuscitation, 231
mucous membrane, 124–125
mucus, 237
multiple sclerosis, 134

nails, 110
necrotizing enterocolitis (NEC), 129
newborn. See baby
nicotine, 222, 223
nipple confusion, 149–151
nipples
  biting, 145
  cramp in small blood vessels, 140–141
  latching on, 21–22, 25–26
  sore, 28–31
noise, 13
Norwegian Medical Association, 155
nursing. See breastfeeding

obesity, 122
ovarian cancer, 216
ovulation, 212
oxytocin
  benefits for mother, 214

cesarean section and, 20, 63
function of, 7
letdown reflex and, 28
in men, 40
nursing time and, 24
scent bonding and, 15
skin contact and, 178
Syntocinon and, 142
womb and, 80

pacifier
  bottle feeding and, 151–152
  limiting use of, 34, 152–153
  milk production and, 147–149
  nipple confusion from, 149–151
  as superstimuli, 151
  teeth position and, 152
painkillers, 53–54, 65
parenting, 250–251
paternal instincts, 7, 10, 39–40
paternity leave, 43–44, 247–248
pediatrician, 99–100
pelvic pain, 87, 96, 208, 214–216
personality changes, 248–249
pethidine, 53–54
phenylketonuria (PKU), 92
phototherapy, 27, 238, 239
physical development, 176–177, 182
PKU (phenylketonuria), 92
placenta, 56, 80–81
plugged milk ducts, 136–137
postnatal contractions, 80
postnatal exercise, 209
postpartum blues, 55–57
postpartum depression, 57–58
postpartum period, 65–66, 97. See also
    mother, postpartum
preeclamptic toxemia, 69
pregnancy, 56, 145, 251–252
premature baby
  breastfeeding, 77–78, 113, 115
  example of, 68
  jaundice and, 238
  necrotizing enterocolitis in, 129
  protein, iron for, 118–119
  sudden infant death syndrome and,
    227
procreation instincts, 40–41
progesterone, 56
projectile vomiting, 242
prolactin, 159, 198
protein, 118–119
psychological development, 179–181, 182
psychosis, 58